Restoring Quality Health Care

SECOND EDITION

Praise for
Restoring Quality Health Care

"Too often, health policy sounds like the secret plan of a mystical cult—arcane, complex, and inaccessible. Scott Atlas is clear, concise, grounded in the facts and a model of elegant simplicity. And it will work!"

> —**DOUGLAS HOLTZ-EAKIN**, former director of the nonpartisan Congressional Budget Office; chief economist of the President's Council of Economic Advisers (2001–02); and current president of the American Action Forum

"Atlas gives us an informed view of how to achieve high quality in health care while bringing costs under control."

> —**GEORGE P. SHULTZ**, Thomas W. and Susan B. Ford Distinguished Fellow, Hoover Institution, Stanford University; and former US secretary of state (1982–89)

"Scott Atlas has written a book that is a must-read for anyone with a serious interest in health policy. Valuable insights and critical information appear on page after page. Read it. You won't be disappointed."

> —**JOHN C. GOODMAN**, president of the Goodman Institute for Public Policy Research

"Improving access and excellence in health care and reducing its costs are core goals for all nations. Scott Atlas articulates with great clarity his original views on key US health system reforms to achieve these goals while preserving innovation to deliver on the promise of twenty-first century medicine."

> —**ELIAS A. ZERHOUNI, MD**, former president of Global Research and Development for Sanofi, a leading global health care and pharmaceutical company; and fifteenth director of the National Institutes of Health (2002–08)

Restoring Quality Health Care

A Six-Point Plan for Comprehensive Reform at Lower Cost

Scott W. Atlas, MD

SECOND EDITION

HOOVER INSTITUTION PRESS

STANFORD UNIVERSITY | STANFORD, CALIFORNIA

With its eminent scholars and world-renowned library and archives, the Hoover Institution seeks to improve the human condition by advancing ideas that promote economic opportunity and prosperity, while securing and safeguarding peace for America and all mankind. The views expressed in its publications are entirely those of the authors and do not necessarily reflect the views of the staff, officers, or Board of Overseers of the Hoover Institution.

hoover.org

Hoover Institution Press Publication No. 713

Hoover Institution at Leland Stanford Junior University,
Stanford, California 94305-6003

First edition, first printing 2016
Second edition, first printing 2020
27   26   25   24   23   22   21   20   8   7   6   5   4   3   2   1

Manufactured in the United States of America
Printed on acid-free, archival-quality paper

Cataloging-in-Publication Data is available from the Library of Congress.
ISBN 978-0-8179-2395-2 (pbk.)
ISBN 978-0-8179-2396-9 (ePub)
ISBN 978-0-8179-2397-6 (Mobipocket)
ISBN 978-0-8179-2398-3 (PDF)

To my father, who often joked,
"My mind's made up,
don't confuse me with the facts."

Contents

List of Figures and Tables

Tables

Preface

The enactment of the 2010 Affordable Care Act (ACA), commonly called Obamacare, catapulted health care reform into a dominant and highly controversial topic among Americans and a hotly contested issue in political campaigns. It is also emblematic of the overall debate in the United States about the role and reach of the US government in public policy. The ACA set forth two fundamental goals for reforming the US health care system: (1) to increase the insured population; and (2) to contain costs by increasing government control over health care. To accomplish these goals, new taxes and unprecedented regulatory authority of the federal government over health insurance and the health care industry were put in place. Its two core elements, a significant Medicaid expansion and subsidies for exchange-based private insurance, were projected to each cost about $850 billion to $1 trillion over the next decade, per Congressional Budget Office analysis. These changes were instituted while disregarding, indeed even doubling down on, the fundamental problems with the existing system—the perverse incentives that caused runaway costs and excluded millions of Americans from accessing the proven excellence of the world's best medical care.

Beyond the notorious broken promises to Americans about keeping their doctors and their insurance plans, the ACA harmed America's health care in demonstrable ways. The ACA did reduce the overall percentage of uninsured, declining from over 17 percent nationally to about 11 percent in recent Gallup polling. However, the bulk of those newly insured under the ACA were millions of low-income Americans funneled into substandard Medicaid coverage, despite the fact that fewer than half of doctors accepted new Medicaid patients, and ignoring the fact that half of doctors with contractual agreements to accept it in practice do not. That refusal of providers to accept Medicaid is not difficult to understand, given that Medicaid pays below the cost of administering the care—doctors and hospitals will not provide care broadly when they lose money per patient served. Even more troubling, Medicaid is widely documented to have worse health outcomes than private insurance, a reality that makes it unconscionable for politicians to celebrate its expansion for the poor.

Even though it is substandard in every meaningful way, expanding Medicaid costs taxpayers greatly. Although thought of as a state-based program, about 60 percent of its financing comes from Federal taxpayers and 40 percent from state budgets, totaling $630 billion in FY 2019. The ACA's extensive regulations also made private insurance unaffordable for many. Premiums for individuals doubled, and they increased for families by 140 percent over four years, even though insurance deductibles (precoverage, out-of-pocket responsibility) also increased substantially. Under the ACA, massive taxpayer dollars were also spent to subsidize private insurance, yet doctor acceptance of that coverage and insurance options for patients worsened dramatically. Almost 75 percent of private plans in ACA insurance exchanges became highly restrictive, with reduced choice of hospitals and specialists. Moreover, the ACA generated a record pace of counterproductive consolidation across the sector, including anticonsumer mergers of doctor practices and hospitals that are generally associated with higher prices of care.

Today, the overall health care debate has substantively changed. In the wake of the ACA's failure to address the system's most important flaws, many former ACA supporters now push for an even more extreme takeover of the US system: overt single-payer health care, or "Medicare for All." Advocates of single-payer care are disregarding established facts and ignoring decades of experience from countries with socialized medicine, as documented in the medical literature and by published statistics from those same governments. Many US political leaders are even proposing to outlaw private insurance, the coverage that over 200 million Americans use. Calls for single-payer health care fail to acknowledge that single-payer systems hold down costs by restricting access to doctors, procedures, technology, and drugs, and those systems have the expected results: worse outcomes, more deaths, and more suffering. With remarkable irony but unreported to Americans, those countries with the longest experience under government-centralized health systems, including the United Kingdom, Sweden, and many others, now use their taxpayer money to pay for private care to remedy their scandalous wait times and poor outcomes.

Health care reform is urgently needed. America's aging population and the growing burden from lifestyle-induced diseases will increasingly require medical care at an unprecedented level. At the same time, we have entered an extraordinary era in medical diagnosis and therapy. Innovative applications of molecular biology, advanced medical technologies, new drug discoveries, and minimally invasive treatments promise earlier diagnoses and safer, more effective cures. Sophisticated "big data" analyses and artificial intelligence (AI) will likely generate new models of personalized health and delivery of care. The possibilities for improving health through technology have never been greater. Yet the current trajectory of the health care system threatens both the sustainability of the system and the essential climate for the innovation necessary to reach this potential.

It is time for a fundamentally different approach to meeting the significant health care challenges facing the nation. *Facts matter, logic matters, and incentives matter.* Instead of framing health care reform as reliant on more government regulation and focusing on reducing the cost of insurance, my plan centers on a completely different paradigm—restoring the appropriate incentives to lower the cost of medical care through competition, based on price and quality, for value-seeking patients. Like other goods and services in the United States, market competition for empowered consumers who control the money would reduce health care costs while increasing its quality. That, in turn, would reduce insurance premiums as well as expenditures from government health programs to accomplish the true goal—broadening access to high-quality health care for all Americans—without restricting access and limiting innovation, faults that are common to all single-payer, centralized systems.

I propose a six-point, strategic, competition-based reform plan for US health care. The foundation of my plan centers on fundamental principles integral to lowering the price of health care while enhancing its value. The plan harnesses the power of patients motivated to seek value, while breaking down anticonsumer barriers to competition among care providers by reducing the government's counterproductive overregulation of health care. It restores the original purpose of health insurance: to protect against the risk of significant and unexpected health care costs. Using specific incentives and targeted deregulation, the proposals detailed in this plan enhance the availability and affordability of twenty-first-century medical care and ensure continued health care innovation. Once this plan is fully implemented, private national health expenditures will decrease by approximately $2.75 trillion over the decade, federal government health expenditures will decrease by approximately $1.5 trillion over the same period, and access to high-quality health care will significantly improve for everyone, especially the poor. These savings will also promote increased activity in other areas of the US economy. And perhaps most important, the health reforms in this plan reflect the key principles held by the American people about what they value and expect from health care in terms of access, choice, and quality.

This book first examines the status of US health care, particularly in light of the ACA. Key data and historical evidence about single-payer health care systems are also noted. Six key reforms central to my competition-based model are then described in detail, each with its underlying rationale, as follows: (1) expand affordable private insurance; (2) establish and liberalize universal health savings accounts (HSAs) to leverage consumer power; (3) instill appropriate incentives with rational tax treatment of health spending; (4) modernize Medicare for the twenty-first century as the population ages; (5) overhaul Medicaid to eliminate the second-tier health system now isolating poor Americans from the excellence of US medical care; and (6) strategically enhance the supply and price transparency of medical care while ensuring innovation.

Setting the Record Straight on US Health Care, Single-Payer Systems, and Medicare for All

The overall goal of US health care reform should be to broaden access for all Americans to high-quality medical care, not to simply label people as "insured." Instead, like today's single-payer rationale, the Affordable Care Act (ACA) aimed first and foremost to increase the percentage of Americans with health insurance. It did so by expanding government insurance and subsidizing heavily ACA-regulated private insurance. Insurance premiums are secondary, though, and chiefly reflect two factors: (1) the cost of medical care, accounting for most of premiums; and (2) the regulatory environment of insurance. Through a series of new regulations, including coverage mandates, co-payment limits, insurance subsidies, and restrictions on medical savings accounts, the ACA counterproductively encouraged more widespread adoption of bloated insurance and furthered the inappropriate construct that insurance should minimize out-of-pocket payment for all medical care. Patients in such plans do not perceive themselves as paying for these services, and neither do physicians and other providers. With patients having little incentive to consider value, prices as well as quality indicators, such as doctor qualifications, remain invisible, and providers don't need to compete. The natural results are overuse of health care services and unrestrained costs.

In response to the failures of the ACA, superimposed on decades of misguided incentives in the system and the considerable health care challenges facing the country, US voters at the time of this writing are being presented with two fundamentally different visions of US health care reform: (1) a single-payer, government-centralized system, including Medicare for All, the extreme model of government regulation and authority over health care and insurance, which is intended to broaden health care availability to everyone while minimizing concern for price; or (2) a competition-based, consumer-driven system, based on increasing competition among providers, removing regulations that shield patients from considering price, and empowering patients with control of the money. This model is intended to reduce the costs of medical care while enhancing its value, thereby providing broader availability of high-quality care for everyone.

Before we consider how to reform the US system to reach the extraordinary promise of twenty-first-century health care, we need to understand the facts about the state of US health care. We also need to examine the data about single-payer nationalized systems.

Background: The Urgency of Reforming America's Health Care System

Health care reform cannot wait. America is facing the greatest health care challenges in its history. Unprecedented demand for costly medical care is a certainty, yet the US already spends significantly more on health care than any other nation.[1] According to the Department of Health and Human Services' Administration on Aging and US Census Bureau statistics, the number of Americans sixty-five and older has increased by a full six million in the past decade alone, to more than 13 percent of the overall population, while those age eighty-five and older have increased by a factor of ten from the 1950s, to today's six million (Figure 1.1).[2] Achieving this goal—longer life spans—paradoxically also means additional health care expenditures. Older people tend to have the most disabling diseases, including heart disease, cancer, stroke, and dementia—the diseases that depend most on specialists, complex technology, and innovative drugs for diagnosis and treatment.

In addition to an aging population, the United States harbors an enormous future disease burden from lifestyle choices, most

FIGURE 1.1. Relative age distribution of total US population, 2010–50 *(top)*; relative age distribution of senior US population, 2020–50 *(bottom)*.

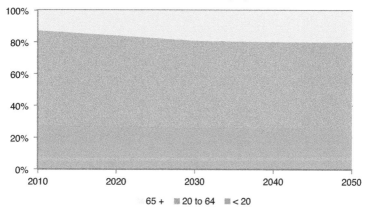

Relative age distribution of total US population, 2010–50

65 +   20 to 64   < 20

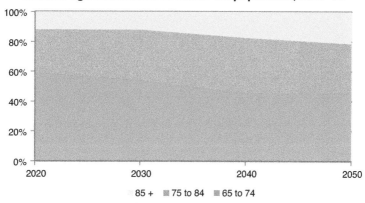

Relative age distribution of senior US population, 2020–50

85 +   75 to 84   65 to 74

The population of seniors is rapidly growing. Among those over sixty-five years of age, the proportions of seniors over seventy-five and over eighty-five are rapidly growing.
Source: US Census Bureau.

notably obesity, smoking, and alcohol abuse. For cancer alone, the most recent US data estimates that 42 percent of all cancers and 45 percent of cancer deaths are attributable to cigarette smoking, excess body weight, and alcohol.[3] Obesity, America's most serious health problem, has increased to crisis levels, already affecting more adults and children in the United States than in any other nation (Figure 1.2).[4] Given the known lag time for such risk factors

FIGURE 1.2. Prevalence of obesity (percent BMI > 30) compared to life expectancy, United States and selected OECD nations.

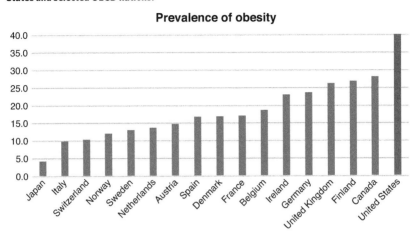

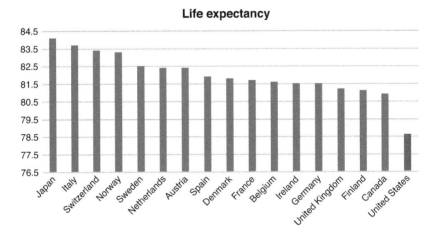

Note the almost direct inverse relationship between life expectancy and the prevalence of obesity. *Source:* Organisation for Economic Co-operation and Development, *OECD Fact Book 2018* (Paris: OECD, 2018).

to impact health, these modifiable lifestyle behaviors threaten unprecedented cumulative health and economic harms over the next several decades.

These daunting demographic realities add to today's already serious fiscal challenges in US health care, which promise to worsen over the near future and overwhelm the system. America's national

FIGURE 1.3. Workers funding Medicare per Medicare beneficiary, historical and projections.

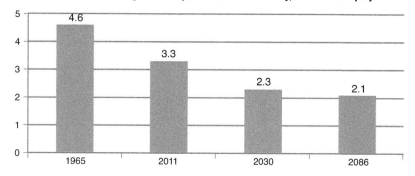

The number of workers per beneficiary supporting Medicare is far less than at the beginning of the program and is rapidly declining.
Source: Centers for Medicare and Medicaid Services, Office of the Actuary, *2014 Annual Report of the Boards of Trustees of the Federal Hospital Insurance and Federal Supplementary Medical Insurance Trust Funds,* July 2014, https://www.cms.gov/research-statistics-data-and-systems/statistics-trends-and-reports/reportstrustfunds/downloads/tr2014.pdf.

health expenditures now total more than $3.8 trillion per year, or 17.8 percent of gross domestic product (GDP), and they are projected to reach 19.4 percent of GDP by 2027.[5] Medicaid, originally covering 250,000 beneficiaries, has expanded to cover more than seventy million people at a cost of over $550 billion per year.[6] Medicare spent less than $1 billion in its first year, but today it spends more than $300 billion annually on hospital benefits alone, and $740 billion in total.[7] In 1965, at the start of Medicare, workers paying taxes for the program numbered 4.6 per beneficiary, whereas that number will decline to 2.3 in 2030 with the aging of the baby boomer generation (Figure 1.3). By 2034, people sixty-five years and older will outnumber children for the first time in US history (77.0 million elderly versus 76.5 million under eighteen), according to the US Census Bureau's National Population Projections. That demographic shift has serious implications.

Outside a discussion of the role of private versus public health insurance is the reality that America's main government insurance programs, Medicare and Medicaid, are already unsustainable unless reformed. The 2019 Medicare Trustees Report projects that the Hospitalization Insurance trust fund will face depletion in 2026.

Regardless of trust fund depletion, Medicare and Medicaid must compete with other spending in the federal budget. Without reforming the current system, federal expenditures for health care and Social Security are projected to consume all federal revenues by 2049, eliminating the capacity for national defense, interest on the debt, or any other domestic program.[8]

Assessing the US Health Care System: A Critical Appraisal

• *The WHO Report*

A decade prior to passage of the ACA, the ambitious *World Health Report 2000* by the World Health Organization (WHO) ranked the health care systems of 191 nations.[9] Its most notorious finding—the relatively low ranking of the United States as thirty-seventh in "overall performance" as defined by the WHO—has been repeatedly asserted by many policy makers and advocacy groups as objective evidence of the overall failure of America's health care, especially in light of the higher expenditure for health care in the United States.

Contrary to initially drawn conclusions from that study, the WHO study methods and conclusions were heavily criticized in a body of peer-reviewed literature by international experts who examined the report in detail. First, almost two-thirds of the WHO rankings were based on *equality* rather than *quality* (Figure 1.4). For instance, a system with C quality but equal performance for everyone would be ranked higher than a system with A quality for some and C quality for others.

Additional serious flaws that undermined the rankings in the report are detailed in the top scientific journals,[10] including (1) highly subjective inputs, many of which do not closely reflect health care access or quality; (2) biased assumptions about the relative importance of inputs; (3) substantial measurement errors; and (4) when data was missing from dozens of countries, it was filled in simply based on assumptions of the study authors. Even the thirty-seventh place overall ranking had already been adjusted downward due to the high expenditure in the United States, rather

FIGURE 1.4. WHO index components.

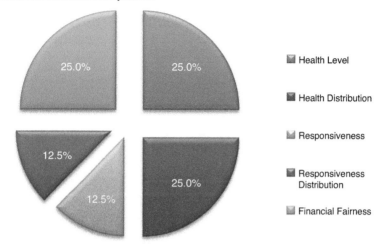

Almost two-thirds (62.5 percent) of a system's overall ranking was based on measures of *equality* rather than *quality*.
Source: World Health Organization, *World Health Report 2000*.

than based on quality per se. Ultimately, Mark Pearson, head of health for the Organisation for Economic Co-operation and Development, the Paris-based organization of the world's largest economies, was quoted as saying, "Health analysts don't like to talk about it (*World Health Report 2000*) in polite company. It's one of those things that we wish would go away."[11]

- *Infant Mortality and Life Expectancy as Indicators of Health Care Quality*

Beyond the widely discredited WHO Report, single-payer advocates often point to America's consistently low ranking in two statistics: *life expectancy* and *infant mortality rate*. But expert studies have proven these two statistics to be grossly flawed in ways that do not reflect health care system quality and also misleadingly rank the United States lower than peer nations.

Consider America's rate of ***infant mortality***—death within the first year after birth—calculated to be 5.9 per 1,000 live births in the latest statistics, thirty-second among thirty-five developed countries, according to the OECD. The most striking flaw is that basic terminology and definitions vary country-to-country, generating false comparisons even among "peer nations." The United States strictly adheres to the WHO definition of live birth ("Irrespective of the duration of the pregnancy . . . breathes or shows any other evidence of life"), counting all births, even extremely premature infants who have the least chance of survival. This isn't true for European nations. The WHO noted that it is "common practice in several countries (e.g., Belgium, France, and Spain) to register as live births only those infants who survived for a specified period beyond birth," and infants who did not survive were completely ignored for registration purposes.[12] A British study of Belgium, Denmark, Finland, France, Germany, Greece, the Netherlands, Norway, Portugal, Spain, Sweden, and the United Kingdom found that terminology alone caused up to 40 percent variation and 17 percent false reductions in infant mortality.[13] Consider this: American physicians consistently make heroic efforts to save extremely premature infants, unlike their counterparts in other countries, who often don't even count such babies when they die. Official data from the US National Center for Health Statistics and the European Perinatal Health Report show that when it comes to newborns who need medical care and have the highest risk of dying, the United States has the world's third-best infant mortality rate—trailing only Sweden and Norway, countries with numerous other significant differences.

Second, premature birth, the main risk factor for infant death, whether from harmful maternal behaviors during pregnancy or other causes, is far more frequent in the United States than any other developed country—65 percent higher than in Britain, more than double that of Ireland and Finland. A Centers for Disease Control (CDC) study found that standardizing for gestational age alone eliminated 68 percent of the difference in infant mortality between Sweden and the United States. The CDC's National Center for Health Statistics concluded, "The primary reason for the United States' higher infant mortality rate when compared with Europe is the United States' much higher percentage of preterm births." [14]

Third, three-fourths of the world's neonatal deaths are counted by highly unreliable household surveys up to five years after pregnancy, instead of being recorded at birth by health care professionals. These surveys frequently misclassify what were really live births as "stillbirths," thereby excluding most neonatal deaths. In the WHO's report *Neonatal and Perinatal Mortality: Country, Regional and Global Estimates,* up to 47 percent of the 192 ranked countries provided unreliable data.[15] The WHO warned that differing mortality rates between countries "may be due to diverging definitions and reporting systems, sources of data, or levels of accuracy and completeness."

America's ***life expectancy*** ranking is also often cited as an indicator of poor-quality health care in the United States. In 2017, life expectancy was 76.1 years for men and 81.1 years for women, twenty-sixth and twenty-ninth, respectively, among the thirty-five developed nations. Yet life expectancy is a coarse statistic that reflects many factors, several of which are wholly unrelated to health care quality (see Table 1.1).

First, life expectancy does not distinguish illness-related death from immediately fatal gunshot wounds or fatal car accidents, deaths that clearly do not reflect health care quality. For those one to twenty-five years of age, two-thirds of US deaths are not from illness; for those twenty-five to forty-four, more than 40 percent are not from illness.[16] For men ages twenty to twenty-four years, accidents and homicides account for 84 percent of the gap in mortality rates between Canada and the United States,[17] with those death rates about six times Sweden's and Canada's, and about ten times those of the United Kingdom and Japan. Just like the distorted rankings from including US neonatal infant deaths that are excluded by other nations, these deaths in younger adults have a particularly significant impact on overall life expectancy calculated from birth, yet they generally do not reflect health care quality.

Second, voluntary, personal lifestyle choices differ among countries and impact life expectancy, but they are not necessarily a reflection of health care quality.[18] Obesity, defined by the OECD

TABLE 1.1. Additional factors influencing the calculations of life expectancy

Lifestyle choices	• Nutritional decisions • Obesity • Exercise or sedentary behavior • Safe-sex practices • Drug abuse • Cigarette smoking • Marriage rates
Population heterogeneity	• Range of genetic predisposition to disease and response to treatment • Range of socioeconomic classes • Range of behaviors acceptable in population subgroups • Income inequality • Education
Societal and environmental conditions	• Homicide rate • Suicide rate • High-speed, fatal motor vehicle collisions • Urbanization
Cultural differences	• Response to behavior recommendations reducing risk for disease • Acceptance of medical advice • Reliability of patients on maintaining doctor-recommended therapies • Willingness to miss work for illness recovery
Differences in decision-based standards of medical care	• Inclusion of all births as recorded live births • Rates of higher-risk multiple births from infertility treatments • Prioritization of preserving high-risk, premature births • Willingness to extend end-of-life care in elderly patients

Many factors influencing the calculation of life expectancy are not related to health care system quality.

as a "non-medical determinant of health," along with tobacco and alcohol consumption, are proven to shorten life expectancy, regardless of country or health care system.[19] Obesity rates are substantially higher in the United States than in any other developed nation. According to the OECD's *Health Statistics 2018*, 40 percent of Americans are obese, compared to 17 percent in France, 13 percent in Sweden, 10.3 percent in Switzerland, 9.8 percent in Italy, and 4.2 percent in Japan, where people have the longest life expectancy. Based on the estimated 6.5 years of lost life expectancy, *obesity differences alone account for approximately 40 percent or more of the life expectancy differences between the United States and almost every other country* (see Figure 1.3).

Life expectancy numbers in the United States are lower, in part, due to a higher historical burden of smoking. Despite declining smoking rates, the United States had the highest level of cigarette consumption per capita over a fifty-year period ending in the mid-1980s compared to all other developed nations.[20] Smoking generally causes death after thirty- to sixty-year lag times, sometimes long after cessation. Life expectancy for smokers is at least ten years shorter than for nonsmokers, according to the CDC. According to the surgeon general, smoking causes 480,000 premature deaths and $300 billion in direct health care expenditures and productivity losses each year in the United States.

Fundamentally, infant mortality and life expectancy calculations are both filled with inconsistencies and inputs unrelated to health care quality—almost all of which deceptively skew the US ranking negatively. The CDC itself explicitly warned at the bottom of its life expectancy table, "Because calculation of life expectancy (LE) estimates varies among countries, ranks are not presented. Therefore, comparisons among countries and their interpretation should be made with caution." [21]

Single Payer and Medicare for All: The Facts

The notion that single-payer health care represents a goal for health system reform is mainly driven by the intuitive attractiveness of a simple concept: the government explicitly "guarantees" medical care. Indeed, many nations claim to "guarantee" health care; many further insist that such health care is provided "free of charge." For instance, the constitutions of the USSR, Venezuela, and many other failed nations with substandard health care under strictly regulated nationalized medical services have had explicit "guarantees" of "free" health care. Today, England's National Health Service Constitution explicitly states, "You have the right to receive

NHS services free of charge"—despite taxing citizens about £125 billion per year, roughly equivalent to $160 billion dollars per year. Canada's "free" health care costs the average family about C$13,311 per year for government health insurance; families among the top 10 percent of income earners in Canada pay C$39,486.[22] Note that Canada's "free" health care actually costs billions of dollars in 2019 to the overall economy and to individuals in forgone wages.[23]

Costs and funding of single-payer health care are often cited as the main objection to its implementation, and there is no question that a nationalized single-payer system would require massive new taxes on working Americans to fund it. The California state senate's 2017 analysis by the Appropriations Committee estimated that the single-payer health care proposed for California alone, SB 562, the Healthy California Act, would cost about $400 billion per year, more than double the state's entire annual budget. Bernie Sanders's current Senate bill to establish single-payer health insurance in the United States, the Medicare for All Act, or M4A, has been estimated to cost over $32 trillion in its first decade. Doubling all currently projected federal individual and corporate income tax collections would be insufficient to finance the added federal costs of the plan.[24] On the other hand, nationalized single-payer systems spend less on health care overall than the United States does. But governments regulate costs in single-payer systems by overtly restricting use. Single-payer systems universally hold down health care costs by limiting availability of doctors, treatments, medications, and technology through their power over patients and doctors as the only direct payer.

The opposition to single-payer care should not focus only on the requirement for massive new taxes, but instead examine the well-documented half century of its failure to provide timely, quality medical care. Single-payer systems in countries with decades of experience have proven to be inferior to the US system in several important objective measures of access to care and quality. The truth is that single-payer systems, including in the United Kingdom, Canada, Sweden, and other European and Nordic countries, impose shockingly long wait times for doctor appointments, diagnostic procedures, drugs, and surgery—wait times that are virtually never found in the United States—specifically as a means to contain costs by rationing care.[25] And that failure to deliver timely medical care has serious consequences, including pain, suffering, and death; worse medical outcomes; permanent disability; lack of patient choice about their own health care; and tremendous costs. Indeed, the Supreme Court of Canada, in the 2005 *Chaoulli v. Quebec* decision, famously stated, "Access to a waiting list is not access to health care."

The consistent failures of single-payer health care to deliver timely care are well documented and include the following:

- ***In those countries with the longest experience of single-payer health care, published data demonstrates massive waiting lists and delays that are unheard of in the United States.*** In England alone, according to government statistics, a record-setting 4.4 million patients are on NHS waiting lists as of October 2019; more than 95,000 have been waiting more than six months for treatment; and more than 4,000 patients have waited more than one full year as of 2019 . . . all *after* already receiving initial diagnosis and referral. As of late 2016, the NHS average wait time exceeded one hundred days for hip or knee replacements, hernia repair, and tonsillectomies. In Canada's single-payer system, the 2017 median wait from general practitioner (GP) appointment to specialist appointment was 10.1 weeks; when added to the median wait of 10.8 weeks from specialist to first treatment, the median wait after seeing a doctor to start treatment was 21 weeks, or about five months.[26] An average wait for a Canadian cardiology patient was 4.9 weeks for the cardiologist appointment after seeing the GP, and another 6.3 weeks to start treatment; that means 11.2 weeks from GP appointment to first treatment. The average Canadian woman waits 10.4 weeks after seeing the GP to see the gynecologist and another 9 weeks to first treatment, or 19.4 weeks total from GP visit to treatment. For simply an appointment with the qualified specialist after

FIGURE 1.5. Median Canadian wait times from GP referral to first specialist treatment.

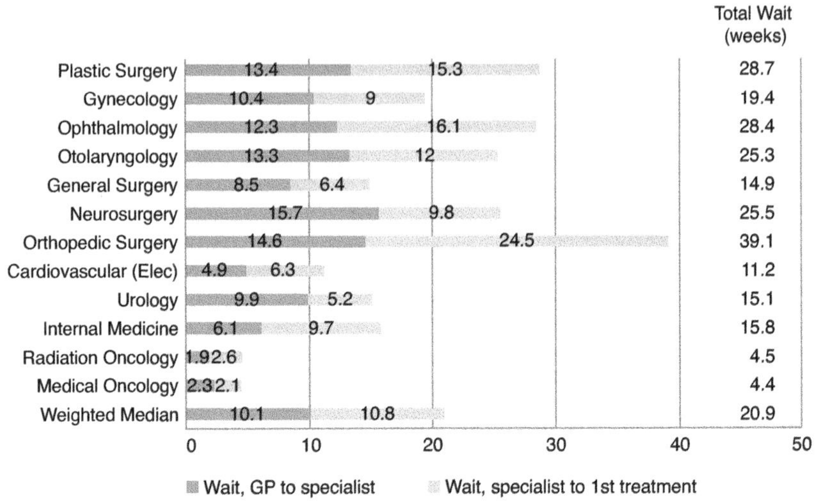

	Wait, GP to specialist	Wait, specialist to 1st treatment	Total Wait (weeks)
Plastic Surgery	13.4	15.3	28.7
Gynecology	10.4	9	19.4
Ophthalmology	12.3	16.1	28.4
Otolaryngology	13.3	12	25.3
General Surgery	8.5	6.4	14.9
Neurosurgery	15.7	9.8	25.5
Orthopedic Surgery	14.6	24.5	39.1
Cardiovascular (Elec)	4.9	6.3	11.2
Urology	9.9	5.2	15.1
Internal Medicine	6.1	9.7	15.8
Radiation Oncology	1.9	2.6	4.5
Medical Oncology	2.3	2.1	4.4
Weighted Median	10.1	10.8	20.9

Canadians face long wait times between seeing their GP and receiving treatment from a specialist. *Source:* Adapted from B. Barua and M. Moir, "Waiting Your Turn: Wait Times for Health Care in Canada," 2019 Report, Fraser Institute.

already waiting and seeing the GP, Canadians wait another 12.3 weeks (three months) for an ophthalmologist; they wait another 15.7 weeks to see a neurosurgeon; and Canadians endure their bone and joint pain for 14.6 weeks (four months) while waiting to see an orthopedist for further evaluation before another 24.5 weeks to treatment (Figure 1.5).

These long waits are characteristic of single-payer systems, but they stand in stark contrast to US health care. Aside from organ transplants, "waiting lists are not a feature in the United States," as stated by the OECD and verified by numerous studies.[27] For instance, Ayanian and Quinn note that "in contrast to England, most United States patients face little or no wait for elective cardiac care."[28] Low-risk patients "sometimes have to wait all day or even be rescheduled for another day," according to the Agency for Healthcare Research and Quality's "Technology Assessment: Cardiac Catheterization in Freestanding Clinics"—that is, a wait for even one single day was considered notable. Ironically, US media reporting was widespread and cited as a wake-up call for whole-system reform when 2009 data showed that time to appointment for Americans averaged 20.5 *days* for five common specialties (note that in 2017, after the implementation of the ACA, wait times had increased by 30 percent compared to 2014).[29] That reporting failed to note that those US waits were for healthy check-ups in almost all cases, by definition the lowest medical priority. *Even for low-priority check-ups and purely elective, routine appointments, US wait times are far shorter than for seriously ill patients in countries with single-payer health care.*

- *In single-payer systems, patients are left waiting months, even after their doctors recommended urgent treatment.* Barua calculates that over a sixteen-year period, more than 44,000 additional Canadian women died due to Canada's wait times for medically necessary nonemergency treatment.[30] In the UK's single-payer NHS, more than 22 percent of those referred for "urgent treatment" for cancer currently wait more than *two months* for their first treatment in England (NHS wait time statistics)—a number that has been increasing despite government efforts, and a number that exceeds even its own arbitrarily set "standard," which declared that it would be acceptable for 15 percent of cancer patients to wait two full months for first treatment (Figure 1.6).

  Similarly, 21 percent of brain surgery patients in England wait more than *four months after diagnosis.* In Canada's single-payer system, the most recent data revealed a median wait for neurosurgery, after already seeing the doctor, of 25.5 weeks—about six months. For their vision-restoring surgery, Canadians with cataracts waited a median time of 20.2 weeks. And in Canada, if you needed orthopedic surgery for severe pain and limited mobility, like hip or knee replacement, you would wait a startling 39.1 weeks.

- *Single-payer systems prevent access to the newest drugs for cancer and serious diseases, sometimes for years, compared to Americans.* Cancer drugs, generally comprising the largest

FIGURE 1.6. Two-month wait from GP "urgent" cancer referral to first treatment.

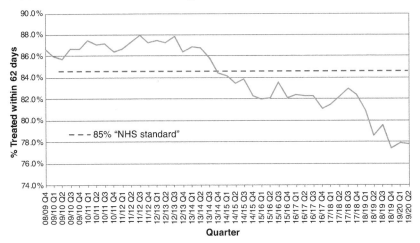

NHS statistics on patient waits for treatment after GP "urgent referral for cancer," past decade through Q2 2019–20.
Source: NHS.

proportion of all new drugs, deserve special consideration, because time is of the essence for treating these life-threatening diseases. OECD data showed that survival is strongly associated with the system's availability of new cancer drugs, specifically more so than the provision of drugs free of charge.[31] The United States has been by far the most frequent location for launching new cancer drugs—by a factor of at least four—surpassing any country studied in the previous decade, including Germany, Japan, Switzerland, France, Canada, Italy, and the UK, according to the *Annals of Oncology*.[32] In a 2011 *Health Affairs* study, the US Food and Drug Administration (FDA) had approved thirty-two of thirty-five new cancer drugs submitted from 2000 to 2011, while the European Medicines Agency (EMA) approved only twenty-six.[33] Median time to approval in the United States was about half that in Europe. All twenty-three drugs approved by both were available to US patients first. Two-thirds of the novel drugs approved in 2015 (twenty-nine of forty-five, or 64 percent) were approved in the United States before any other

FIGURE 1.7. Availability of the world's new cancer drugs by country, within two years after 2013–17 launch (as of December 2018).

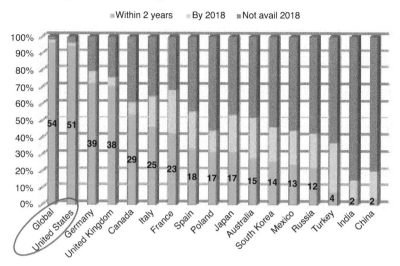

Source: IQVIA Institute, *Global Oncology Trends 2019: Therapeutics, Clinical Development and Health System Implications,* 2019; data via *Statista,* https://www.statista.com/statistics/696020 /availability-of-new-oncology-drugs-by-country. Exact number of drugs available in each country of the world's total of 54 is noted; green shaded column in chart indicates percentage of the 54 total.

country.[34] Compared to American women, who had access to twenty-six new hormonal contraceptive drugs over a fifteen-year period, women in single-payer Canada and in the UK had far fewer choices (62 percent and 54 percent, respectively), as reported in the Canadian medical literature in 2016.[35]

Of all newly approved cancer drugs from 2009 to 2014, single-payer systems of the UK, Australia, France, and Canada had only approved 30–60 percent of those approved in the United States by June 30, 2014.[36] The latest data shows that of the world's fifty-four new cancer drugs launched from 2013 to 2017 and available within two years, fifty-one (94 percent) were available within two years in the United States (Figure 1.7).[37] For Brits with cancer, only thirty-eight of fifty-four (70 percent) were available; for Canada's cancer patients, only twenty-nine of fifty-four (53 percent) were available; cancer patients in France had access to only twenty-three of fifty-four (43 percent); and Australian cancer patients had access to fifteen of fifty-four (28 percent).

And yet, in 2017, single-payer NHS England introduced a new "Budget Impact Test" to cap drug prices specifically based on expenditures rather than medical efficacy.[38] This will further restrict drug access, even though cancer patients could be forced to wait years for life-saving drugs, some dying as they wait for drugs already available in the United States. As just one important projection under that single-payer NHS rule, a dementia drug for Alzheimer's disease would have to cost only £29.60/year, less than US$4 per month, or it would be unavailable to patients (as calculated by the Alzheimer's Society), ironically restricted due to overall cost to the system specifically because so many patients need it.

- *Single-payer systems cannot outperform the US system even in something as scheduled as routine cancer screening tests.* Confirming numerous prior OECD studies, Howard reported in 2009, before ACA requirements, that the United States had superior screening rates compared to all ten European countries with nationalized systems (Austria, Denmark, France, Germany, Greece, Italy, the Netherlands, Spain, Sweden, and Switzerland) for all cancers.[39] Likewise, Canada's single-payer system fails to deliver screening tests for the most common cancers, including PAP smears, colonoscopy, and PSA tests, as widely as in the US system.[40] And compared to Europeans, Americans are more likely to be screened for cancer younger, when the expected benefit is greatest. Not surprisingly, US patients have less advanced disease at diagnosis than in Europe for almost all cancers.

Long waits in single-payer systems for diagnosis, treatment, drugs, and technology have major consequences to patients, as documented throughout the peer-reviewed medical journals using data, not anecdotes. The ultimate consequence of single-payer care is worse health outcomes compared to the US system for nearly all of the most serious diseases—the illnesses that cause the most

FIGURE 1.8. Comparison of five-year survival rate, United States versus Western Europe, 2000–2002, from seven common cancers.

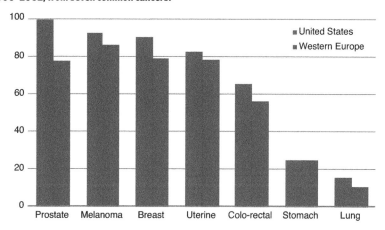

The United States has superior survival from all common cancers compared to western European nations.

Source: A. Verdecchia et al., "Recent Cancer Survival in Europe: A 2000–02 Period Analysis of EUROCARE-4 Data," *Lancet Oncology* 8(9) (2007): 784–96.

FIGURE 1.9. Comparison of five-year survival rates for men and women, United States versus Western Europe.

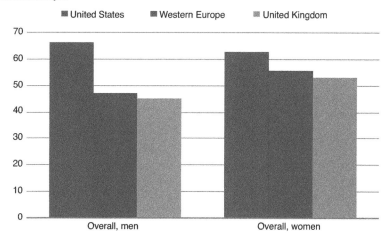

Note the statistically significant increased survival for American men and women compared to the average Western European, and especially the UK.

Source: A. Verdecchia et al., "Recent Cancer Survival in Europe: A 2000–02 Period Analysis of EUROCARE-4 Data," *Lancet Oncology* 8(9) (2007): 784–96.

FIGURE 1.10. High blood pressure: access to treatment (*top*) and successful control (*bottom*). Percentage of treated patients by country, ages thirty-five to sixty-four years.

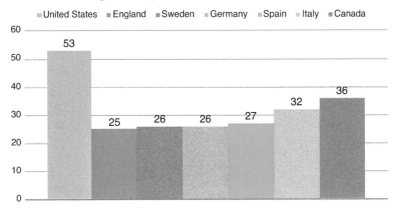

High blood pressure: access to treatment

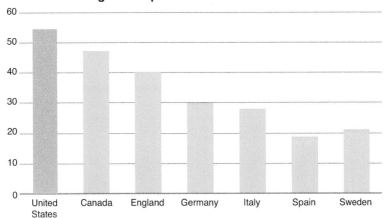

High blood pressure: successful control

The United States has more effective medical care for high blood pressure compared to other developed countries, including those held as models for single-payer care.
Source: K. Wolf-Maier et al., "Hypertension Treatment and Control in Five European Countries, Canada, and the United States," *Hypertension* 43(1) (2004): 10–17.

deaths and the most important chronic diseases that lead to the most disability and death,[41] including cancer,[42] heart disease,[43] stroke,[44] hypertension,[45] and diabetes[46] (Figures 1.8, 1.9, 1.10). *Why should Americans voluntarily move toward a system that has proved worse than current US health care?*

What Should We Learn from Countries with Long-Standing Single-Payer Systems?

Americans should also ask why the United States would move toward single-payer care when countries all over the world with decades of single-payer experience now turn toward private health care to solve their failures. Even though England's NHS is projected to hit a £30B funding shortfall in 2020–21, one of the very few areas where funding is increasing is to non-NHS providers. In one year alone, £901 million targeted for medical services by the UK government (half of the total increase) was used to buy care from private and other non-NHS providers.[47] Sweden, often heralded as the paradigm of a successful welfare state, has failed its citizens in health care access. To fix their system, Swedish municipal governments have increased spending on private care contracts by 50 percent in the past decade. Primary care clinics and nursing facilities are now run by the private sector or receive substantial public funding. Private sector competition has also been introduced into Sweden's pharmacies to tear down the previous government monopoly on prescription and nonprescription drugs. Since 2007, Denmark's patients using taxpayer-funded single-payer health care can choose a private hospital in or outside the country if the waiting time for the treatment exceeds one month.[48] *Governments of Finland, Ireland, Italy, the UK, the Netherlands, Norway, Spain, Sweden, and Denmark, all with single-payer care, now spend taxpayer money on private care, sometimes even outside their own country, to solve their unconscionable failures to deliver adequate care.*

Americans should wonder why people with financial means would need to spend even more money than their already high taxes for something that is "guaranteed and free." After all, who wouldn't want "guaranteed, free health care"? The answer is found in existing single-payer systems all over the world that offer those same "guarantees." People with the financial means increasingly choose to circumvent their single-payer systems for private health care. Even though they already pay the equivalent of $160 billion dollars per year for their single-payer NHS, half of all Brits who earn more than £50,000 buy or plan to buy private health insurance, according to *Statista 2017*. In Sweden, about 650,000 who can afford it buy private insurance despite already paying $20,000 per family per year through taxes for their nationalized system, according to *Insurance in Sweden 2015*. And over 250,000 Brits spend out-of-pocket cash for private care, despite paying over US$4,200 per person per year in taxes for their NHS. According to the European insurance and reinsurance federation (CEA), private insurance in the EU bought by those who can afford it grew by more than 50 percent over a decade to 2010, specifically to fill the "ever growing gaps in coverage" in public health systems. *Here is the reality: only the poor and the middle class are stuck with nationalized, single-payer health care, because only they cannot afford to circumvent that system.*

Medicare for All: Creating Our Own Single-Payer Program?

Those who advocate a conversion to Medicare for All fail to acknowledge the widely published historical evidence in the world's top medical journals on existing single-payer systems in countries with decades of experience. Single-payer systems all over the world have proven to be inferior to the current US system in virtually every important objective measure of care, including less access to care and inferior quality of care, resulting in worse outcomes from virtually all serious diseases. And that should not be a surprise. Single-payer systems hold down health care costs by limiting availability of doctors, treatments, medications, and technology. And they are able to do so through their dominant power over patients, most of whom do not have the financial means to circumvent the system.

Our own government's Medicaid and Medicare programs employ similar methods to hold down costs. Data on payments to health care providers shows a significant underpayment from both Medicare and Medicaid for health care services (Figure 1.11). That

FIGURE 1.11. Underpayment to hospitals for delivered care, Medicare and Medicaid, 2004–17.

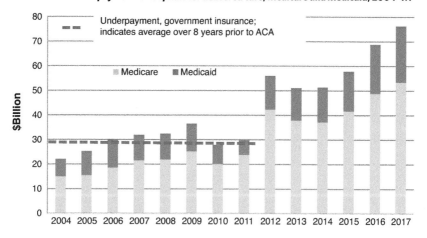

Note the significant jump in the deficit to hospitals from payment *below cost* of services by government insurance after ACA regulations came into effect.
Source: Analysis of American Hospital Association Annual Survey data, 2018, community hospitals.

underpayment—payment for services *below the cost* of administering those services—has increased significantly since the implementation of the ACA. This underpayment has consequences beyond shifting costs to those with private insurance.

Studies throughout the medical literature demonstrate that outcomes under Medicaid, where most patients are limited to purely government insurance with its restrictive coverage, are worse than those for medically similar patients under private coverage (Table 1.2).

And Medicare for All advocates fail to acknowledge that access to care is *already at risk* under today's Medicare due to below-cost payment for care (CMS Office of the Actuary, J. Shatto and M. K. Clemens, April 22, 2019). The Office of the Actuary of the Centers for Medicare and Medicaid Services (CMS) in 2019 has warned of serious limitations in availability of care for Medicare beneficiaries. CMS calculated that most hospitals, skilled nursing facilities, and in-home health care providers already lose money per Medicare patient. Specifically, CMS warned that "we expect

TABLE 1.2 Comparison of disease outcomes, Medicaid patients versus privately insured patients.

Medical Disorder	Comparison to Private Insurance and No Insurance
Major surgery	Need longer hospital care (42% longer), incur more hospital costs (26% more), and almost two times more likely to die in the hospital than those with private insurance; 13% more likely to die, stayed in the hospital 50% longer, and care cost 20% more than those with NO insurance (LaPar et al., *Ann Surgery* 2010; 893,658 major surgeries)
Cancer of the mouth and throat	50% more likely to die than patients with private health insurance (Kwok et al., *Cancer* 2010; 1,231 patients)
Colon cancer	57% more likely to die postoperatively compared with patients with private insurance, a death rate not significantly different from the uninsured (Kelz et al., *Cancer* 2004; 13,415 adults)
Heart procedures	More likely to have strokes and heart attacks and die than patients with private insurance and suffered the same outcome as those who lacked insurance altogether; more than twice the risk of death, heart attack, or other serious cardiac event within one year of cardiac surgery compared to privately insured patients (Gaglia et al., *Am J Cardiology* 2011; 13,573 patients)
Lung transplants	Die sooner than patients with private insurance undergoing lung transplants for end-stage pulmonary diseases; 8.1% less likely to survive ten years after surgery than privately insured and uninsured patients (Allen et al., *J Heart Lung Transpl* 2011; 11,385 patients)

Even after standardizing for medical differences among patients, Medicaid patients fare worse than those under private insurance, sometimes even worse than those with no insurance at all.

access to Medicare-participating physicians to become a significant issue in the long term under current law."

Americans should also understand what is obvious but hidden in discussions by single-payer advocates. Medicare for All or any other single-payer system would almost immediately jeopardize their medical care, and it's even documented in the proposals themselves.[49] The text of the Medicare for All bill necessitates large and immediate reductions in payments to doctors and hospitals now treating patients under private insurance, including cuts of more than 40 percent for hospitals and 30 percent for physicians, with these cuts growing more severe over time. As Blahous states, we cannot know with certainty the extent to which these cuts would disrupt the supply and timeliness of health care services. With certainty, though, we know that public insurance for all will mean less access to doctors, procedures, drugs, and technology, just like in all other single-payer systems, in addition to closures of hospitals and clinical practices. Asserting that the access and quality Americans enjoy today, with their private insurance or private coverage supplements to Medicare, would be maintained if everyone used Medicare and private insurance were abolished, is fantasy at best. *Ironically, Medicare is already unsustainable, even without expanding it.*

Despite today's vilification of private insurers, Medicare ranks at or near the top for the highest rates of claim refusals—*more than nearly all comparison private insurers every year* on the AMA Insurer Report Card. Even in their current limited form, our own single-payer systems are already fraught with problems, including errors, fraud, and waste. Our own Veterans Administration single-payer system needed to turn to private care to remedy its inadequacies, through the extended and broadened Veterans Choice Program in 2017. Medicare throws away $60 billion of taxpayers' money per year, by Government Accountability Office estimates.[50] The Office of the Inspector General reported in 2018 that "California made Medicaid payments of $738.2 million ($628.8 million Federal share) on behalf of 366,078 ineligible beneficiaries and $416.5 million ($402.4 million Federal share) on behalf of 79,055 potentially ineligible beneficiaries."[51]

And here is another unacknowledged truth: more than 70 percent of US seniors choose to rely on private insurance to supplement or replace traditional Medicare coverage.[52] *Why would beneficiaries need that if purely government insurance was already so satisfactory?*

The Public Option as a Pathway to Single Payer

What's wrong with offering government insurance as an "option" without a requirement to switch? Government insurance expansions mainly erode, or "crowd out," private insurance, rather than provide coverage to the uninsured. MIT professor and Obamacare adviser Jonathan Gruber showed that when government insurance expands, the number of privately insured falls by about 60 percent as much as the number of publicly insured rises.[53]

Consider the experience in Hawaii. Only seven months after offering Keiki Care in 2008, the country's only statewide universal child health insurance, the state ended the program. In fact, over 80 percent of those taking up the program already had private insurance. And with that shift, massive new costs were shifted from those previously paying for their own private insurance onto other taxpayers.

Premiums for private insurance will further skyrocket because of underpayment by government insurance compared with costs of services. According to the American Hospital Association, the nearly $60 billion underpayment by Medicare and Medicaid surged to an all-time high, nearly doubling, once Obamacare's regulations came into play. Even before the ACA, it was calculated that a family of four with private insurance paid an extra $1,512 per year in private premiums, and an extra $1,788 per year for all health expenses (insurance, co-pays, and deductibles).[54] This adds a significant burden for families paying private premiums, and expanding that will make private insurance even more expensive.

Why would people switch from private insurance to public insurance? Public insurance is typically cheaper, because public insurance restricts coverage for care and pays less to providers—in fact, even below the costs of delivering the care—which results in even less access to medical care and even less choice of providers for patients. This is already proven worldwide.

The public option is not a moderate or compromise proposal—it is simply a slower, more insidious pathway to single-payer health care for nearly everyone. The death of affordable private insurance is the inevitable consequence of a single-payer option. Indeed, even those Democratic candidates calling for a public option openly admitted in the presidential debates that such an option will inevitably lead to single-payer for all. By introducing the public option, private insurance would disappear for all but the affluent, the only people who could afford that choice. And America's health care would become even more divided, as in the UK, Sweden, and elsewhere, where only the lower and middle classes suffer the full effects of inferior single-payer care.

Conclusion

US health care demands reform. Health care costs are unsustainable and increasing, and that high cost already leaves some people, particularly the poor, isolated from the proven excellence of US medical care. Contrary to their false guarantees, government-centralized single-payer systems hold down health care costs mainly by strictly limiting the use of important medical care, drugs, and technology, through their power over patients and doctors as the payer. By the data in the medical literature, single-payer health care has been proved, worldwide, to be inferior to the US system, with severe costs far beyond massive tax increases. And make no mistake about it: America's most vulnerable, the poor and the middle class, will undoubtedly suffer the most if the system turns to single-payer health care, because only they will be unable to circumvent that system.

We know there is an alternative approach, but it is not easily encapsulated into a marketing slogan. The critical concept is that *reducing the cost of medical care by competition* is the most effective pathway to broader access to quality care, lower insurance premiums, and ultimately better health. Instead, most post-ACA ideas continue to stress making *insurance* more affordable, either through cash to consumers in refundable tax credits or other subsidies, or now by instituting government-run single-payer care. Insurance premiums are only secondary, though, and historically chiefly reflect two factors: (1) the cost of medical care, accounting for about 80 percent of insurance premiums; and (2) the regulatory environment, accounting for most of the rest.

Rather than compelling Americans to accept an inferior government-run system that universally restricts access to important drugs, technology, and medical care to regulate costs, let's focus on creating conditions long proven to bring down prices while simultaneously improving quality in virtually every other good or service in America. History shows that the best way to control prices and improve quality for all goods and services is through competition for empowered, value-seeking consumers. Positioning patients, including seniors, as direct payers while financially rewarding them for seeking value with their money would stimulate competition among doctors and hospitals. Reducing the price of health care by competition, instead of more regulation, will lower insurance premiums, reduce outlays from government programs, and broaden access to quality care for everyone. Broadly available options for cheaper, high-deductible coverage less burdened by regulations; markedly expanded health savings accounts; and tax reforms to unleash consumer power are keys to achieving price sensitivity for health care. Coupling those with strategic increases in the supply of medical care by breaking down anticonsumer barriers to competition and transparency of price and quality among doctors and hospitals would generate competition and reduce the price of health care. These reforms would permit all Americans, rich or poor, to access the same excellence of medical care that the affluent, including the most strident advocates of single-payer care for the rest of us, all use for their own health care.

CHAPTER TWO

Reform #1:
Expand Affordable Private Insurance

Principal Features of Reform #1: Expand Affordable Private Insurance

- Permit all insurers (on or off any state or federal exchanges) to offer true high-deductible, limited-mandate catastrophic coverage (LMCC) plans to all citizens, covering hospitalizations, outpatient visits, diagnostic tests, prescription drugs, and mental health.
- Transfer ownership of coverage to the individual so that it is portable, leaving the employer still available for sign-up and automation of payments.
- Permit insurers to eliminate Obamacare's 3:1 age-based premiums.
- Permit insurers to risk-adjust premiums for obesity, as is already allowed for smoking.
- Eliminate the health insurance premium excise tax.

The Importance of Private Health Insurance

Private insurance is a core part of the excellence of US health care. Beyond the 175 million Americans under age sixty-five who use private insurance for their health care, roughly 70 percent of Medicare beneficiaries today also utilize private insurance to supplement or replace traditional Medicare coverage, whether Medicare Advantage, Medi-Gap, and employer-sponsored coverage, and millions more use private drug coverage. Moreover, patients on pure government insurance depend on reimbursements to providers from the privately insured to subsidize their medical care.

First, broad access to doctors and hospitals comes with private insurance, not government insurance. Categorizing someone as "insured" is not the same as enabling timely, quality health care for them. The harsh reality awaiting low-income Americans thinking that expansion of the program automatically equals access to care is that most doctors already refuse to take new Medicaid patients, in numbers that dwarf the percentage refusing to take new private insurance patients, and this was the case well before the Medicaid expansion, because of government-defined low reimbursements (i.e., below costs of delivering care).[1] According to a 2017 Merritt Hawkins report, only 53 percent of doctors in major metropolitan areas continue to accept Medicaid.[2] The Department of Health and Human Services (HHS) reported that even of those providers signed by contract and on state lists to provide care to new Medicaid enrollees, 51 percent were not available to new Medicaid patients.[3] This is especially true of general/family practice doctors, psychiatrists, and pediatricians, all of whom accept Medicaid patients at far lower rates than they accept patients with private insurance.[4] That refusal of providers to accept Medicaid is solely due to lack of adequate payment. Medicaid pays below the cost of administering the care, and doctors and hospitals will not provide care broadly when they lose money per patient served.

A superficial look at Medicare acceptance appears satisfactory, but on scrutiny we see a different scenario unfolding today. Just as a massive part of the US population ages into Medicare eligibility, a growing proportion of doctors do not accept Medicare patients. In a 2014 physician survey, about one-quarter of doctors no longer see Medicare patients or limit the number they see; in primary care, 34 percent refuse Medicare patients.[5] More recently, the average rate of Medicare acceptance among physicians in the fifteen major metro markets surveyed by Merritt Hawkins was 84.5 percent and 81 percent for midsize markets. Even in 2015, only 72 percent accepted *new* Medicare patients, significantly fewer than those accepting privately insured new patients.[6] Historically, few doctors opted out of Medicare, with that number first hitting triple digits in 2010, at 130. But those numbers jumped from 130 in 2010, before ACA regulations, to over 1,600 in 2013, and spiked at 7,400 in 2016.

The trend slowed to 3,732 in 2017, to now total over 25,000, according to CMS data.[7]

Beyond simple acceptance of Medicare insurance by doctors and hospitals is the financial reality of sustainable access for beneficiaries. CMS calculates that most hospitals, skilled nursing facilities, and in-home health care providers already lose money per Medicare patient. CMS's Office of the Actuary warned in 2019 of serious limitations of availability of care for Medicare beneficiaries in the immediate and longer-term future. CMS stated, "We expect access to Medicare-participating physicians to become a significant issue in the long term under current law"[8]—regardless of any change in Medicare eligibility.

Second, beyond access to care, the quality of medical care is also superior with private insurance. Studies throughout the medical literature demonstrate that outcomes under Medicaid, where patients are generally limited to purely government insurance with its restrictive coverage, are worse than those for medically similar patients under private coverage. That quality difference for the privately insured includes fewer in-hospital deaths, fewer complications from surgery, longer survival after treatment, and shorter hospital stays than similar patients with government insurance.[9] Restricted access to important drugs, specialists, and technology for those using government insurance most likely accounts for these differences.

Third, America's hospitals and providers depend on the higher payments from private insurance for solvency. Just like government insurance in single-payer systems, our own government's Medicaid and Medicare programs hold down costs by paying less for care. The actuary for CMS calculates that Medicare and Medicaid pay roughly 60 percent of what private insurance pays for inpatient services, and about 60 to 80 percent for physician services. But that's only part of the story. While private insurance pays over 140 percent of the cost of care, Medicare and Medicaid pay *less than cost*. That underpayment gap—payment for services below the *cost* of administering those services—has increased significantly since implementation of the ACA. The Office of the Actuary of CMS in 2018 calculated that most hospitals, skilled nursing facilities, and in-home health care providers already lose money per Medicare patient. CMS predicts that by 2040, approximately half of hospitals, two-thirds of skilled nursing facilities, and over 80 percent of home health agencies will be operating at a loss, even without any change toward single payer, due to the influx of Medicare beneficiaries with the aging population. Rural hospitals, in particular, are more vulnerable to closure, since they have a significantly smaller proportion of patients with private insurance. *Without private insurance, the access and quality of care Americans enjoy today under any government coverage will greatly diminish.*

The Harmful Impact of the ACA on Private Insurance

The ACA has had a harmful impact on private health insurance. As a direct result of the ACA's new regulations on pricing and its new mandates on coverage, the law has already forced millions of Americans off of their existing private health plans. The Congressional Budget Office (CBO) projected that a stunning ten million Americans will be forced off their chosen employer-based health insurance by 2021—a tenfold increase in the number that was initially projected back in 2011.[10] Meanwhile, private insurance premiums have greatly increased under Obamacare. In its first four years, ACA private insurance premiums for individuals doubled and increased for families by 140 percent; this occurred even though insurance deductibles (the amount that must be paid before services are covered by the plan) for individuals increased by over 30 percent for individuals and by over 97 percent for families (Figure 2.1).[11] As time passed, insurance options and prices on ACA exchanges continued to worsen, according to the Department of Health and Human Services.[12] Many exchange enrollees continued to face large year-on-year premium increases in 2018, according to Kaiser Foundation analysis, even in the face of markedly higher deductibles.[13]

The shift to government insurance itself also increases private insurance premiums. Because government reimbursement for

FIGURE 2.1. Impact of ACA regulations on private insurance premiums and deductibles, first four years.

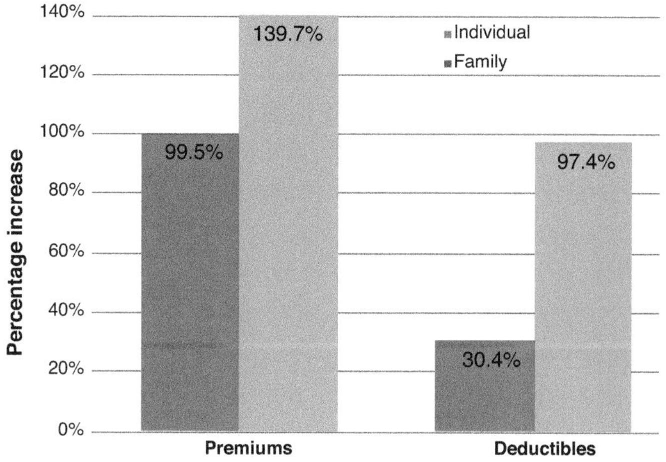

Source: eHealth, January 2017 data.

health care is below cost, costs are shifted back to the privately insured, pushing up premiums. In some calculations, the under-payment by government insurance adds $1,800 per year to every family of four with private insurance.[14] Nationally, the gap between private insurance payment and government underpayment has become the widest in twenty years, doubling since the initiation of Obamacare.[15]

Choices of private insurance and providers covered under them are dwindling as well, despite the theory that the law would increase insurance choices and competition. According to a December 2014 study, the exchanges offer 21 percent fewer plans than the pre-Obamacare individual market, with a decrease to 310 nationally in 2015 compared to 395 insurers in the individual market in 2013, the last year before implementation of Obamacare.[16] For 2018, only one exchange insurer offered coverage in approximately one-half of US counties. As the CBO stated, "Insurance premiums are lower in markets with more insurers, because insurers have stronger incentives to keep premiums low."[17] This rise will impact not only the individual paying the premiums but also taxpayers, because taxpayers subsidize those increasing premiums under Obamacare. Note that the federal government (i.e., federal taxpayers) subsidizes most private premiums—directly or indirectly—at a cost of roughly $300 billion in fiscal year 2016.

For middle-income Americans dependent on subsidized private insurance through government exchanges, the ACA has eliminated access to many of the best specialists and best hospitals. McKinsey reported that 68 percent of those policies cover only narrow or very narrow provider networks, double that of the previous year.[18] The majority of America's best hospitals in the National Comprehensive Cancer Network were not covered in most of their states' exchange plans. Under Obamacare insurance plans, analysis showed a severe shortage of the specialists essential to diagnosing and treating stroke, one of the most disabling and lethal diseases in the United States (in some cities, the number is actually down to zero).19 Almost 75 percent of ACA private plans became "highly restrictive," with far fewer hospitals, primary care doctors, and specialists accepting that insurance.[20]

Keys to Expanding Affordable Private Insurance

Fundamental change to private insurance is vital to maximizing patient access to quality health care while leveraging consumer power and expanding health care access for everyone, including those on government assistance. The ACA has made private insurance less affordable and pushed health insurance reform in the wrong direction. Strategies to subsidize premiums artificially prop up mandate-filled insurance coverage that typically minimizes out-of-pocket payment. This is directly counterproductive, because it shields patients from caring about price, and medical care providers from competing on value. It encouraged more widespread adoption of bloated insurance and furthered the erroneous view that insurance should minimize direct payment by patients and subsidize the entire gamut of medical services, including routine medical care. When that inappropriate function of insurance is combined with the cloak of secrecy shielding health care prices and provider qualifications, consumers have neither an incentive nor the necessary means to incorporate value into health care decisions. The natural results are inappropriate use of health care services and unrestrained costs.

On the other hand, high deductibles with catastrophic coverage would restore the essential purpose of insurance—to reduce the risk of incurring large and unanticipated medical expenses. Because they would pay for most medical care directly, consumers would have the incentive to choose wisely. Provider prices would consequently become more visible and align with what consumers value, rather than being set artificially or by government decree.

The behavior of American consumers counters the ACA's approach to insurance reform and validates the argument that higher-deductible coverage both generates more affordable insurance and reduces health spending. First, consumers choose to buy high-deductible coverage and choose higher deductibles when offered those plans. In over a decade since the tracking of this type of coverage, consumers have increasingly selected high-deductible plans (Figure 2.2). Among those enrollees, a shift toward higher deductibles has continued, with a tripling of those consumers with deductibles over $3,000 since the ACA was passed (Figure 2.3).[21] Second, consumer spending on health care is significantly lower for those using high-deductible coverage,[22] without any consequent increases in emergency room visits or hospitalizations and without the hypothesized harmful impact on low-income families or the chronically ill.[23] Health spending reductions averaged 15 percent annually, and the savings increased with the level of the deductible and when paired with HSAs. More than one-third of the savings by enrollees resulted from lower costs per health care utilization,[24] that is, value-based decision-making by consumers. Additional evidence from studies of consumers' use of magnetic resonance imaging (MRIs) and outpatient surgery shows that introducing price transparency and defined-contribution benefits further encourages price comparisons by patients.[25] While especially relevant to patients

FIGURE 2.2. Percentage of covered employees with a deductible of $2,000 or more, single coverage, by firm size and year.

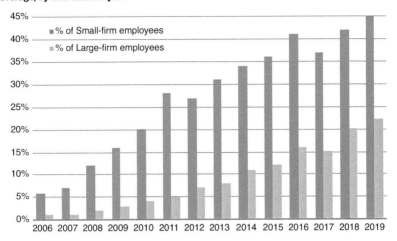

Consumers have increasingly chosen high-deductible coverage, although the increase has slowed.
Source: Data compiled from Employer Annual Health Benefits surveys, Kaiser Family Foundation, http://kff.org/health-costs/report/employer-health-benefits-annual-survey-archives.

FIGURE 2.3. Deductible distribution in high-deductible plans with savings account options, by year.

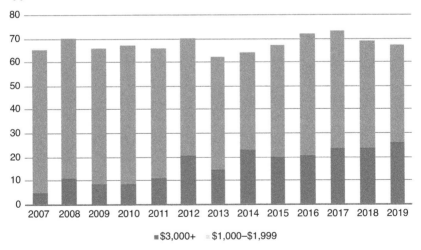

Among those enrolled into high-deductible coverage, consumers have shifted to higher deductibles.
Source: Data compiled from Employer Annual Health Benefits surveys, Kaiser Family Foundation, http://kff.org/health-costs/report/employer-health-benefits-annual-survey-archives.

FIGURE 2.4. Growth rate increases in HDHPs have slowed since ACA passage.

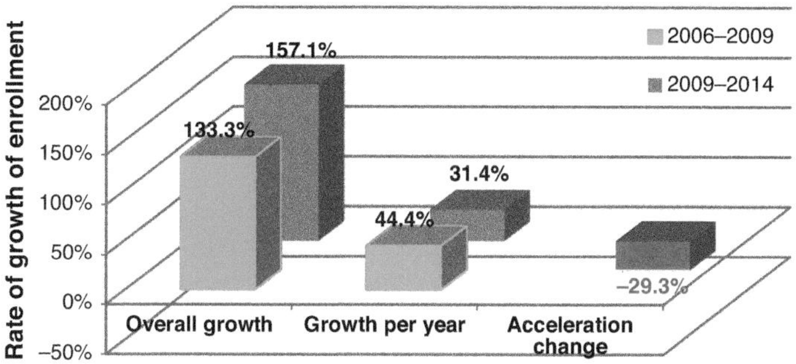

Enrollment Rate of Growth, Deductible of $2,000+; Single Coverage, All Firms, Pre- vs. Post-ACA Bill Passage. Although high-deductible plans are still growing as a choice for consumers, the rate of increase slowed under the ACA.
Source: Data compiled from Employer Annual Health Benefits surveys, Kaiser Family Foundation, http://kff.org/health-costs/report/employer-health-benefits-annual-survey-archives.

using high-deductible plans with HSAs, these reforms would reduce expenditures by all health care consumers.

Affordable private insurance has been increasingly the choice for Americans, specifically with high deductibles and HSAs. Making both of those options more available should be a principal focus of health care reform, particularly because that combination ultimately results in decreasing health care prices for everyone, including those using other forms of coverage. To expand affordable private insurance options, we need to reduce several counterproductive regulations on insurance, many of which have specifically harmed high-deductible plans. While consumers are still increasingly opting for plans with deductibles greater than $2,000, the growth rates slowed once ACA mandates and restrictions were implemented (Figure 2.4). In addition, the premiums of high-deductible plans accelerated faster after the passage of the ACA than any other coverage (Figures 2.5 and 2.6), although they remain less costly than the other types of coverage.[26] We cannot be certain whether these changes are entirely caused by Obamacare regulations, such as limits on deductibles and mandated coverage, but health system reforms should not selectively make these plans less affordable for consumers. Restoring the choice of

FIGURE 2.5. Premiums by plan type, before and after passage of the ACA.

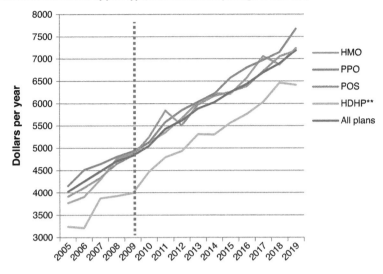

The annual premiums (single coverage) for all types of insurance coverage have continued to increase over the decade since the ACA (vertical line indicates passage of ACA bill).
Notes: HMO, health maintenance organization; *PPO*, preferred provider organization; *POS*, point of service; *HDHP*, high-deductible health plan. Premiums include both employee and employer payments.
**HDHP includes high-deductible plans offered with either a health reimbursement arrangement or an HSA.
Source: Data compiled from Employer Annual Health Benefits surveys, Kaiser Family Foundation, http://kff.org/health-costs/report/employer-health-benefits-annual-survey-archives.

limited-mandate coverage with truly high deductibles would create the more affordable coverage that many consumers value and increasingly seek.

We should eliminate unnecessary coverage mandates that have ballooned under the ACA, so consumers could opt for more tailored, cheaper coverage that they deem a better value for their money. Let's strip back many of Obamacare's so-called minimum essential benefits, which have increased premiums by almost 10 percent, and eliminate most of the more than 2,270 state mandates requiring coverage for everything from acupuncture to marriage therapy.[27] We should remove archaic obstacles to competition, including barriers to out-of-state insurance purchases. To eliminate unfair cost shifts imposed by the ACA that raised premiums

FIGURE 2.6. Acceleration of high-deductible health plan premium increases (%) before (2005–09) vs. after (2009–14) passage of ACA.

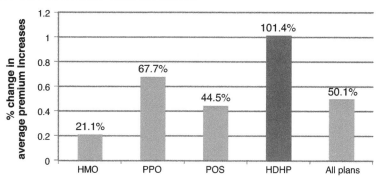

Although all types of insurance plans have increased in price faster after the bill's passage compared to before the bill's passage, Obamacare regulations immediately accelerated the increase in premiums of high-deductible plans more than any other type of coverage.
Notes: HMO, health maintenance organization; *PPO,* preferred provider organization; *POS,* point of service; *HDHP,* high-deductible health plan. The high-deductible plans include those offered with either a health reimbursement arrangement or an HSA; premiums include both employee and employer payments.
Source: Data compiled from Employer Annual Health Benefits surveys, Kaiser Family Foundation, http://kff.org/health-costs/report/employer-health-benefits-annual-survey-archives.

for younger, healthier enrollees by 19–35 percent, we should remove the 3:1 ACA dictate on actuarial regulations for age-rated premiums.[28] Finally, if not enacted by the time of this publication, we should repeal the ACA's annual health insurance providers fee ($11.3 billion in 2015), which insurers pass on to enrollees through increased premiums, according to the CBO.[29] The ACA imposed this sales tax on health insurance beginning in 2014, and the Joint Committee on Taxation (JCT) estimated that the tax burden will exceed $100 billion over its first decade and raise consumers' premiums by up to 3.7 percent per year. This specific tax will increase insurance costs by thousands of dollars over the decade for individuals, families, businesses, and even beneficiaries of the government's own insurance programs—both Medicare and Medicaid.[30]

In addition, health insurance reform is an opportunity to incentivize healthy lifestyles by smart deregulation, rather than more government intervention. Two behaviors deserve special consideration. Cigarette smoking and obesity are the two most important lifestyle behaviors, both proved to increase the risk for highly morbid chronic disease and worsen outcomes from those diseases, regardless of health care quality. The most recent US data estimates that 42 percent of all cancers and 45 percent of cancer deaths are attributable to cigarette smoking, excess body weight, and alcohol.[31] Smoking causes $193 billion in direct health care expenditures and productivity losses each year, according to the Centers for Disease Control.[32] Extra medical care for obesity alone accounts for up to 10 percent of total US health care costs.[33] Because of obesity's high prevalence and its association with multiple chronic diseases, worse treatment results, and more complications from even the best care, the annual US societal costs of obesity exceed $215 billion.[34] While smoking has declined, the burden of obesity to the US health care system and to taxpayers has increased to crisis levels. This situation will only increase over the coming decades, given that diseases from these risk factors typically show a lag time of decades. Even without a reduction, some of the costs could be alleviated. Eric Finkelstein of Duke University has projected that "*keeping obesity rates level could yield a savings of nearly $550 billion in medical expenditures over the next two decades.*"[35] Health care reform in the United States urgently needs to embrace a new era of personal responsibility, and obesity, American society's most serious current public health problem because of both its costs and its damage to people's health, should be the highest priority.

Just as in other types of insurance, premiums that reflect the higher risk of disease and more frequent use of medical care as a consequence of voluntary high-risk behavior are sensible, especially because three-fourths of health insurance claims may result from lifestyle choices.[36] Life insurance premiums are markedly higher for dangerous behavior such as smoking. Risky driving is a key factor in determining automobile insurance rates. Obesity and smoking are high-risk lifestyles, both of which are major drivers of health expense with well-known health hazards. A 1998 study showed that claims of individuals with a high body mass index (BMI) cost $3,537 (2015 dollars) more per year than claims of individuals with low BMI.[37] A 2012 study showed that annual medical costs for people who are obese were $1,429 higher in 2006 than those for people of normal weight; for Medicare patients, this difference was $1,723, with almost 40 percent the result of extra prescription drugs.[38] These numbers exceed the extra medical costs from smoking. A growing number of employers charge smokers higher insurance premiums. In the individual insurance market, the "obese BMI" category paid 22.6 percent more in premiums, and those with "overweight BMI" paid 12.8 percent more than "normal BMI" enrollees.[39] While acknowledging the complexity of and limited knowledge about the influence of genetics on obesity development as well as the harmful health effects of obesity in any individual, actuarially based premium differences for obesity should be allowed in all health insurance plans.

CHAPTER THREE

Reform #2:
Establish and Liberalize Universal Health Savings Accounts

Principal Features of Reform #2: Establish and Liberalize Universal Health Savings Accounts

- Automatically open health savings accounts for every citizen with a Social Security number (or at birth).
- Allow every individual, including seniors, to own a health savings account immediately.
- Make all accounts fully portable, fully controlled by the individual.
- Permit the employer to still serve as center for sign-ups and automated contributions to accounts.
- Eliminate the HSA eligibility requirement for specific deductibles in accompanying insurance coverage.
- Allow significantly higher contribution maximums to equal those of total annual out-of-pocket limits.
- Permit broader uses for spending (health care products and services; use by family members).
- Ease limits on employer-provided financial incentives for wellness programs.
- Allow tax-free rollovers of all health savings accounts to all surviving family members.

The Rationale for Health Savings Accounts

Although health savings accounts (HSAs) can be key to expanding affordable, quality care, HSAs are poorly understood by both advocates and critics. Independent HSAs allow individuals to set aside money tax free for *uncovered expenses*, including routine care. Both contributions and disbursements from the HSA are tax free as long as they are spent on allowable health care. Tax deductions or income exclusions introduce incentives that subsidize health care spending relative to other spending. HSAs have two important distinguishing features different from tax deductions alone: they reward saving, and they position patients to directly buy their own health care. Valuable HSAs introduce a strong incentive to seek value, based on both price and quality, into an individual's decision to buy health care. This stimulates competition among doctors and hospitals, which generates lower prices and better value for *all* patients.

Two key points are essential to clarify from the start, in order to fully understand the role and importance of HSAs in US health care reform:

- *The HSA is a vital and highly effective tool to broaden access to affordable, high-quality health care for all Americans, even those without HSAs.* It does so by putting consumers directly in charge of buying their own health care. The fundamental purpose of an HSA is NOT simply to provide a tax-sheltered benefit for individuals, in order to cushion the blow of high health care expenses; instead, the purpose is to maximize the downward pressure on price of care using the power of motivated consumers.
- *The HSA is not an isolated, independent component of the health care system.* Rather, HSA optimization is intimately related to other aspects of the health care system, including insurance structure and regulation, tax policy, and the supply of providers.

But is it realistic to suggest that patients could seriously consider price and value as they seek medical care? Only 6 percent of health care expenditures are for emergency medical care.[1] Among privately insured adults under age sixty-five, almost 60 percent of all health expenditures is for elective outpatient care.[2] Even in the elderly, almost 40 percent of expenses are for outpatient care. For the top 1 percent of spenders, the group responsible for more than one-quarter of all health spending, a full 45 percent of spending is

FIGURE 3.1. Enrollment in HSAs since introduction, by year.

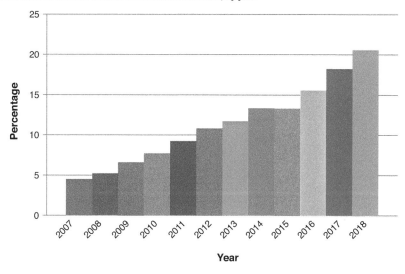

Source: CDC/National Health Care Surveys, National Health Interview Surveys, 2007–18, Family Core component.

also for outpatient care. Nonemergency, scheduled services dominate America's health spending, and therefore they are amenable to price-conscious purchasing.

Despite the ACA's attempt to shift consumers to bloated coverage, a move toward high-deductible plans with HSAs has continued. Indeed, American consumers are approving their value by increasingly choosing HSAs when given the opportunity (Figure 3.1). The percentage of persons enrolled in a HSA with high-deductible coverage almost tripled, from 7.7 percent in 2010 to 20.6 percent in the first nine months of 2018.[3] The total number of HSAs grew to 25 million at the end of 2018, up 13 percent from one year previously.[4] Note that this is not a "tax shelter for the rich"—median household income for HSA holders is $57,060; two-thirds earn less than $75,000 a year.[5] By increasingly choosing HSAs when given the opportunity, American consumers are approving their value. This endorsement by Americans is particularly striking when considering the declining enrollment—from 85.1 percent in 2007 to 56.6 percent in 2017—in traditional coverage, as chosen by employed adults.

Nearly one-third of all employers now offer some type of HSA, up from just 4 percent in 2005, including 62 percent of firms with more than 1,000 employees and 56 percent with 200–999 workers. HSA account holders contributed almost $33.7 billion to their accounts in 2018, up 22 percent from the year before. Devenir projects that, by the end of 2020, HSA total assets held will approach $75 billion in approximately 30 million accounts. Beyond representing an option for more affordable private insurance, pairing HSAs with high-deductible coverage has been shown to reduce the cost of health care—the most effective way to broaden access to quality care without restricting its use. Adding HSAs to high-deductible plans provides stronger incentives to save than other coverage; in Haviland's 2011 study, adding HSAs to high-deductible plans correlated to an increased savings of from 5.5 percent to 14.1 percent, that is, 50 percent higher to more than double the savings from high-deductible plans alone.[6] System-wide health expenditures would fall by an estimated $57 billion per year if only half of Americans with employer-sponsored insurance enrolled in plans combining HSAs with high deductibles.[7] Savings would increase further if deductibles were truly high—for example, $5,000 or more, and if these plans were freed from the added, costly mandates of the ACA. Total savings from these reforms could approach $2 trillion over the decade.

How to Optimize the Impact of Health Savings Accounts

The fundamental point is that HSAs, especially when combined with high-deductible coverage, incentivize and leverage the power of consumers. As in every other good or service in the United States, consumer power is crucial to making health care more affordable while maintaining health care excellence, access, and innovation. Widespread HSAs, when paired with cheaper high-deductible plans, could pay for the bulk of all medical care events, since most health care involves smaller, noncatastrophic expenses. The more people are positioned to pay directly for more of their care, the more downward pressure on prices will occur through providers competing for cost-conscious patients. *The issue is not whether these accounts are effective; it is how to maximize their adoption and eliminate the government rules that serve as obstacles to their use.*

The first step is to elevate the value of HSAs to account holders and make them more widely available. One important step would be to automatically open (but not fund) an HSA for every citizen with a Social Security number or at birth. To maximize consumer leverage on prices, full HSA participation by all citizens, specifically including seniors, should be allowed. Given that seniors are the biggest users of health care, motivating them to seek value is a crucial part of exerting downward pressure on health care prices. All HSAs should be independently owned by individuals, eliminating more restrictive variants that are tied to specific employers. HSAs should be delinked from any specific insurance deductible requirement, a counterproductive regulation that limits HSA participation. That requirement also eliminates the possibility of HSAs with more tailored insurance plans. The only requirement for making contributions to the newly configured HSA should be that the enrollee has active catastrophic insurance coverage, without any specified deductible. These changes would broaden the eligibility for HSAs, so more consumers would be equipped with the tools and incentives necessary to consider price and value when seeking health care.

The second step is to enhance the value of the HSA for the account holder. We should immediately liberalize maximum contributions to the level of total annual out-of-pocket expenses under the ACA (for 2020, $8,150 for individuals and $16,300 for families). Restrictions on HSA use should be eased, most importantly for the expenses of the HSA holder's elderly parents and other family members, regardless of formally defined economic dependency on the account holder. And the list of allowable health care services and products that can be purchased with HSA funds should be expanded. Account rollovers to any surviving family member, not just spouses, while maintaining a tax-sheltered status should be permitted.

TABLE 3.1. Health savings accounts, selected current versus proposed regulations.

Criterion	Current HSA	New HSA
General eligibility	Must meet specific requirements	Universal for all citizens; automatically opened at birth
Insurance requirement to contribute to HSA	High-deductible coverage, deductible level specified by federal government. For 2020: $1,400 (individual) $2,800 (family)	Catastrophic coverage (no other specific requirement; no specified deductible range)
Limits on maximum contribution per year	$3,550 (individual) $7,100 (family) (2020)	$8,150 (individual) $16,300 (family) (matches 2020 ACA max out-of-pocket)
Uses of HSA funds	Not for nonprescription drugs other than insulin	• Over-the-counter drugs are eligible without need for a prescription • Usable for parents, children, siblings, spouse
Tax deductibility	Contributions and withdrawals deductible	Contributions and withdrawals deductible
Eligibility if enrolled in Medicaid	Not eligible, unless exemption	Eligible
Eligibility if enrolled in Medicare	Not eligible	Eligible

The differences between current regulations and this plan's proposed new rules for HSAs are summarized in Table 3.1 (also see "Key Questions and Answers on the Atlas Plan" for further details).

HSAs can also serve as a valuable vehicle through which employers offer health-related benefits, like wellness programs and screening tests (e.g., blood pressure, body mass index, and cholesterol). Although benefits from these programs have been inconsistently demonstrated, more than 90 percent of employers offered lifestyle programs in 2015,[8] increasing from 73 percent in 2011 and 57 percent in 2009 in one source. Most firms offering health benefits in 2019 offer programs to help workers identify health risks and unhealthy behaviors. Among firms offering health benefits,

TABLE 3.1. (continued)

Criterion	Current HSA	New HSA
Eligibility if receiving Social Security?	Not eligible	Eligible
Special Medicare Advantage MSAs	List of restrictions limiting contribution levels, contribution sources, others	Full conversion to standard HSA; no special limits or restrictions
Penalty for ineligible withdrawals	20% penalty (plus taxation)	50% penalty (plus taxation)
Uses for insurance premiums (seniors only)	Can reimburse for money withheld from Social Security to pay Medicare Part B (e.g., $104.90/mo for 2015); can make tax-free HSA withdrawals for Medicare Part D, Medicare Advantage premiums (not Medigap).	Allowed for all premiums
Seniors and ineligible withdrawals	After age 65, taxation	After age 70, 20% penalty
Transfers into HSAs from retirement accounts	Not allowed	Allowed without penalty for seniors
Tax treatment to beneficiary on death of HSA holder	If spouse, tax-free rollover into HSA; otherwise, taxable income	If any family member, tax-free rollover into HSA

26 percent of small firms and 52 percent of large firms offer workers the chance to complete a biometric screening that measures risk factors, such as body mass index (BMI), cholesterol, blood pressure, stress, and nutrition. Fifty-eight percent of large firms with biometric screening programs offer workers an incentive to complete the screening, such as gift cards; lower employee premium contributions or cost sharing; and financial rewards, such as cash or contributions to HSAs. Half of small firms and 84 percent of large firms offer a program in smoking cessation, weight management, or lifestyle coaching.[9] Of the 41 percent of large firms offering incentives for participation, 16 percent have a maximum incentive of $150 or less, while 20 percent have a maximum incentive of more than $1,000.

Many employers now provide overt financial incentives to employee participants. These include lower insurance premiums (57 percent of employers), reduced cost sharing, and higher employer contributions to individual HSAs (34 percent of employers).[10] Significant gains in productivity, marked reductions in health claims, improvement of chronic illnesses, and major cost savings have been shown in some studies, although inconsistently demonstrated, and some have benefited both participant employees and their employers.[11] Medical costs and absentee day costs fall by about three to six dollars for every dollar spent on some wellness programs.[12] The ACA limits the financial incentives from employers, including cash deposits into employee HSAs, to 30 percent of the cost of that employee's health coverage. Abolishing that arbitrary limit would expand these potential motivators for employees to participate in screening and tailored wellness programs.

CHAPTER FOUR

Reform #3:
Instill Rational Tax Treatment of Health Spending with Appropriate Incentives

Principal Features of Reform #3: Instill Rational Tax Treatment of Health Spending with Appropriate Incentives

- Make tax treatment of health expenses universal, that is, equal for all, whether individual, self-employed, or employer-based.
- Allow income tax and payroll tax exclusions for only two categories of expenses:
  - limited-mandate catastrophic insurance premiums
  - HSA contributions for those with catastrophic insurance coverage.
- Base income exclusion on new maximum HSA contribution (equivalent to the total annual out-of-pocket maximum).
- Index income exclusion increases to the Consumer Price Index for All Urban Consumers (CPI-U).

The income tax subsidy for unlimited health spending is one of the great mistakes of modern US tax policy. It creates harmful incentives for consumers that are counterproductive to competition and pricing, it replaces higher wages, and it is regressive, preferentially giving high-income earners more tax breaks.

Tax preferences for health care spending began as a somewhat unintended tax policy, arising from the fact that pension and health insurance fringe benefits provided by employers were not subject to wage controls imposed during World War II to maintain war production.[1] Later, employer payments for health benefits became deductible to employers and tax-excluded to employees in the Internal Revenue Service tax code.[2] The current tax code sets no limits on this income exclusion, contrary to the original intent of Congress in 1954.[3]

The largest tax subsidy for private health insurance—the exclusion from income and payroll taxes of employer and employee contributions for employer-sponsored insurance—cost approximately $280 billion in lost federal tax revenue in 2018, by CBO estimates. In addition, the federal tax deduction for health expenses (including premiums) exceeding 10 percent of adjusted gross income is estimated to cost $12.4 billion in lost tax revenue in 2014.[4] The CBO projects that tax expenditure for employment-based insurance (including income and payroll taxes) will remain close to 1.5 percent of GDP during the coming decade.[5] The tax subsidy is highly preferential to individuals with higher incomes, that is, it is highly regressive. About 85 percent of the subsidy goes to individuals in the top one-half of the income distribution.[6] In addition, the tax exclusion distorts the labor market by limiting job mobility and strongly influencing retirement decisions.[7] Still, certain positives come from employer-sponsored insurance, such as convenience of enrollment, risk pooling, and the employees' opportunity to select insurance for more than one year at a time.

Beyond the numbers, the current tax exclusion creates perverse incentives. Indeed, the observation that "the tax subsidy is responsible for much of what is widely perceived as a health care crisis" may sound like it was written only recently, yet this statement dates back almost forty years.[8] The exclusion makes health spending seem less expensive than it is. The incentive to allocate more money for health care encourages more expensive insurance policies with more elaborate coverage as well as higher demand for medical care regardless of cost. CBO estimates that the income exclusion subsidizes approximately 30 percent of premiums. The current tax exclusion is preferential to insurance over out-of-pocket spending (as opposed to the incentive of HSAs, particularly as structured in this reform proposal). The distortion of health insurance to its now-dominant form, which covers almost all billable services, including minor, fully predictable medical care, while minimizing direct payment by patients, is partly attributable to the tax preference. This preference has greatly increased the overall cost of health care.[9]

Changing the tax treatment of health spending is an important part of urgently needed health care reforms; unfortunately, comprehensive tax reform that would result in a broad-based, low-rate, simple system seems unlikely at this time. Removing the existing tax exclusion entirely would be problematic.[10] Serious repercussions could include a significant increase in the number of uninsured, an abrupt disruption of the labor market, and a dramatic increase in taxes.

Given those realities, the tax reform proposed herein eliminates the Obamacare excise tax and incorporates three main features: (1) universality regardless of the source of health benefits; (2) limits on the total allowed exclusion and; (3) new criteria on eligible spending for tax exclusion, limited only to HSA contributions and premium payments for limited-mandate catastrophic coverage (LMCC). These tax reforms would reduce expenditures and encourage value-based insurance purchasing, that is, they would realign incentives in health insurance and health care markets to benefit consumers. Once the reforms are enacted, the increase in the individual's purchasing power for medical care more than compensates for the loss of certain tax subsidies for health care spending. Each reform is discussed in more detail below.

Universality of Tax Preferences

The current system preferentially benefits higher-income earners who receive health benefits from employers. Current law permits families without employer-based health insurance to deduct medical expenses only if they itemize their deductions, a strategy chosen far more frequently by upper-income earners; moreover, the deduction is limited to expenses that exceed 10 percent of adjusted gross income. To level the playing field, I propose that all citizens be allowed the same deductibility of health expenses if they purchase the basic LMCC. The proposed income exclusion for health spending will be applicable to all, regardless of employment or source of health benefits.

Total Allowable Exclusion Limit

The proposed allowable exclusion from income and payroll taxes is based on the maximum allowable HSA contribution ($8,150). For 2019, the estimated annual health insurance premium paid per worker equaled $7,188 for individual coverage; the average premium paid for high-deductible coverage equaled $6,412. Still, the term "high deductible" was defined as plans with annual deductibles only greater than or equal to $1,350 for an individual ($2,700 for a family); it also included coverage bloated by all of the ACA mandates and regulations. In the final year before ACA regulations, 2009, the average premium of high-deductible plans equaled 82.6 percent of the average cost of employer-provided health insurance, based on annual surveys of employer health benefits. Therefore, given other reforms in this six-point proposal that would further reduce the cost of true high-deductible coverage, the new exclusion should cover the entire cost of high-deductible plans plus significant deposits to HSAs.

The CBO and the JCT estimate that setting income exclusion limits on the basis of the fiftieth percentile for health insurance benefits paid by or through employers in 2015 (and indexed in subsequent years for inflation using the CPI-U), with the same limits for the deduction for health insurance available to self-employed people, would reduce the deficit by $537 billion over the next decade.[11] This cap would have a far greater impact on upper-income earners.[12] (Note, for contrast, that the Urban Institute estimated that capping the exclusion at the seventy-fifth percentile of total health benefit through employment would produce $264 billion in new income and payroll tax revenues over the coming decade.[13]

Eligible Spending for Income Exclusion

Current health spending eligible for tax exclusion is both unlimited in size (until the delayed ACA "Cadillac tax" implementation; see below for more on this tax) and essentially unlimited in the scope of eligible expenses. My proposal would add incentives for purchasing basic catastrophic coverage, beyond limiting the amount of the income exclusion and in addition to other incentives already described. Excludable health spending will apply only to two health expenses: (1) deposits to HSAs; and (2) premium payments for high-deductible, limited-mandate catastrophic coverage. It would be counterproductive to subsidize and incentivize the purchase of insurance bloated with expensive coverage requirements that minimize co-pays and effectively eliminate concern about price of care. Added insurance coverage, including more expensive "comprehensive" coverage, will always be available to those who wish to purchase it.

Employees should also be permitted to purchase their health care coverage directly—that is, outside the limited choices offered by employers—and still maintain the same tax preference, as proposed by Herzlinger and Richman.[14] This would allow many individuals to choose from a larger list of insurance choices (in my plan, only limited-mandate catastrophic coverage), given that 75 percent of insured employees in large firms and 91 percent in small firms had a choice of only one or two plans.[15] Assuming that some of these plans would be less expensive than those provided directly through employers, the employee should be able to receive the excess "health benefit" as taxable income. Note that current law treats all such income to employees as taxable, even if it is used for health insurance. Beyond adding competition and ultimately reducing the price of care, Herzlinger and Richman calculate that under current law (i.e., without my proposed changes described elsewhere in this proposal), this change would allow after-tax household income to grow substantially and payroll tax revenues to increase by $39 to $163 billion per year.[16]

Note that my plan also replaces the changes to the current tax exclusion under Obamacare set to begin in 2022. Under the ACA, a new excise tax (known as the "Cadillac tax") is set to be imposed on employment-based health benefits whose total value—including employers' and employees' tax-excluded contributions for insurance premiums and contributions made through health reimbursement accounts, flexible spending accounts, or HSAs for other health care costs—is greater than specified thresholds (subsequently to be indexed to the growth of the CPI-U). The JCT and the CBO project that those thresholds will be $11,200 for single coverage and $30,150 for family coverage in 2022. The excise tax will equal 40 percent of the difference between the total value of tax-excluded contributions and the threshold beginning in 2022. But designing a policy whereby a government imposes new taxes on products whose prices became unnecessarily high directly because of the government's policies is not only bad for consumers but frankly absurd. Moreover, the Cadillac tax is set to include contributions that employers and individuals make to HSAs toward the thresholds for invoking the 40 percent excise tax. This is a classic example of a misguided government intervention harming an excellent consumer-oriented program (HSAs and high-deductible plans), ironically penalizing individuals trying to lower their health expenses.

CHAPTER FIVE

Reform #4:
Modernize Medicare for
the Twenty-First Century

Principal Features of Reform #4: Modernize Medicare for the Twenty-First Century

- Introduce more options for private insurance for all Medicare enrollees by competitive bidding, along with strong incentives for beneficiaries that add lower cost coverage.
  - Define the benefit as premium support, calculated from a regional benchmark average price of three lowest-priced approved plans.
  - Include limited-mandate, high-deductible coverage as one of the three plans determining the benchmark average.
  - Require all plans defining the calculated benchmark to include prescription drug benefits.
  - Set benchmarks using market-based premiums.
  - Permit beneficiaries to choose breadth of coverage, rather than requiring extensive coverage.
  - Provide full cash rebates directly to beneficiary's newly permitted HSA (not to the plan or to Medicare) if the beneficiary chooses a plan with a premium less than benchmark; require payment from enrollees if premiums of chosen plan exceed benchmark.
- Establish expanded HSAs for all Medicare enrollees.
  - Automatically open an account for every Medicare enrollee; *limits and uses match other HSAs.*
  - Convert current HSA variants under Medicare to new HSAs.
  - Permit tax-free rollovers of all HSAs to any surviving family member.
- Include catastrophic coverage program (annual out-of-pocket limits) in all Medicare plans.
- Phase out taxpayer subsidies for high-income-earning seniors.
- Modernize eligibility to reflect today's demographics, with gradual phase-in to age seventy.

Medicare is a complex program targeted at the elderly, who have already at least partially paid tax contributions over the years for their future health care insurance. Originally, Medicare was put forward as a safety net for protecting senior citizens from financial ruin by catastrophic illness. A key rationale for Medicare was that the program would enable seniors to avoid financial dependence, as evidenced by their lower incomes. This thinking ignored the fact that senior citizens had more substantial assets than younger adult populations during the years of the passage of the Medicare bill.[1] Even more ironic, original Medicare never had—and even today, traditional Medicare still does not include—catastrophic insurance for asset protection.

Today's Medicare is highly fragmented, almost undecipherable in its complexity, flawed in its coverage, and inadequate in its benefits. After decades of coverage additions and patchwork remedies, today's Medicare is a confusing amalgam of four relatively separate insurance programs, each with complicated and diverse funding sources.

- *Part A* (hospital insurance) covers inpatient services, some home care, skilled nursing services, and hospice care. It is funded through the federal payroll tax by today's working population and employers. Most people do not pay a premium for Part A because they (or a spouse) have already paid via their payroll taxes while employed, although they do pay deductibles and co-payments.
- *Part B* (medical insurance) covers doctor bills, outpatient treatment, screening and lab tests, and certain medical supplies, subject to deductibles and co-payments. It is funded partly by beneficiaries via income-adjusted monthly premiums and partly by general tax revenues.
- *Part C* (Medicare Advantage, or MA) is a private insurance system that includes Part A and Part B benefits (i.e., it replaces Parts A and B, so-called traditional Medicare coverage), as well as some prescription drug coverage, for regional beneficiaries. As opposed to traditional Medicare, MA plans must have annual out-of-pocket limits (i.e., catastrophic coverage). In MA,

Medicare contracts with private insurers to offer health services through a variety of provider networks, almost two-thirds
of which are health maintenance organizations (HMOs). MA is
funded partly by member premiums and partly by capitated
payments from taxpayer funds (note that since 2006, Medicare
has paid plans under a bidding process, whereby Medicare
receives bids from private insurers for coverage equal to Parts A
and B and then pays the insurer for coverage relative to formu-
laic benchmarks by county or region).

• *Part D* (prescription drug coverage) is funded by income-adjusted
enrollee premiums and taxpayer funds, as is Part B; co-payments
and deductibles vary by plan. In Part D, private insurance companies provide the coverage. Beneficiaries choose the drug plan
and pay a monthly premium.

In addition to this enormous programmatic complexity, Medicare administrators process nearly 4.9 million Medicare claims each
business day, according to CMS. Unsurprisingly, the Medicare
program is fraught with errors, fraud, and waste, estimated by
the Government Accountability Office to have totaled $60 billion
in 2014.[2]

*Regardless of its intent, or even its flawed coverage, Medicare
must be changed to save it for elderly Americans.* Today and in the
immediate future, timely access to care under Medicare is under
severe pressure, even without moving toward a Medicare for All
system. Owing to the level of Medicare payments for care, most
hospitals and other providers lose money per patient served under
this program. Even under the unlikely scenario of maintaining
today's levels of payments for services, the Office of the Actuary of
CMS in 2019 already warned of serious limitations of availability
of care for Medicare beneficiaries. CMS calculated that approximately 80 percent of hospitals now lose money treating Medicare
patients; by 2040, approximately half of hospitals, two-thirds of
skilled nursing facilities, and over 80 percent of home health
agencies would lose money overall, even with continued profit

from private insurance collections. CMS stated that "we expect access to Medicare-participating physicians to become a significant issue in the long term under current law." And despite today's vilification of private insurers, Medicare ranks at or near the top for the highest rates of claim refusals—more than nearly all comparison private insurers every year on the AMA Insurer Report Card.

Despite its below-cost payments to health care providers, Medicare is in serious financial trouble, even without expanding eligibility, as many propose (also see chapter 1). Beyond the projection in the 2019 Medicare trustees report that the Hospital Insurance Trust Fund will be depleted in 2026 is the issue of the funding base for the program. Just as the population of seniors is dramatically expanding, the taxpayer base financing the program is dramatically shrinking. Those individuals funding benefits—that is, taxpaying workers per beneficiary—have declined by half since program inception. In its first year, Medicare spent under $1 billion for 250,000 senior citizens, but today it spends over $740 billion for more than 70 million enrollees. Nearly four million Americans now reach age sixty-five every year. In 2050, the sixty-five-and-over population is projected to reach double the number in 2012. And the future health care needs for seniors have dramatically increased. The already high health expenses for a sixty-five-year-old (Figure 5.1) will triple by 2030.[3] Americans live 25 percent longer after age sixty-five now than in 1972,[4] with an average life expectancy of about eighty-five years, approximately five years longer than at the inception of Medicare (Figure 5.2). With longer life come more health care needs. Today's seniors need to save money for decades, not just years, of future health care.

Although patients may not know it, traditional Medicare overtly limits the choice of doctors by virtue of its complex restrictions and rules about accepting "assignment" of Medicare insurance. "Assignment" means that a doctor has agreed to accept the Medicare-approved amount as full payment for services. Doctors who formally opt out can charge patients whatever they want, but they must forgo

FIGURE 5.1. Per capita health care expenses, by age.

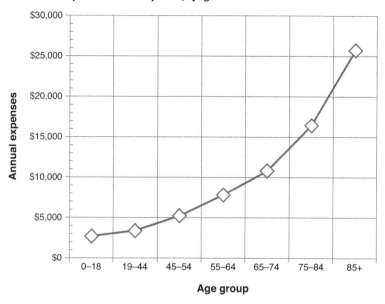

Age is a clear predictor of health care utilization and health care costs per person.
Source: Centers for Medicare and Medicaid Services (2014).

FIGURE 5.2. Additional years of life expectancy in the United States for sixty-five-year-olds, 1965–2038.

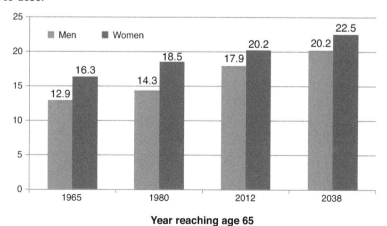

The additional life expectancy for those already reaching sixty-five years of age (top of each column) has increased greatly since 1965, when Medicare began.
Source: CDC/National Center for Health Statistics, *National Vital Statistics Reports* 62, no. 7 (January 2014).

filing Medicare claims for two years, and their Medicare-eligible patients must pay out of pocket to see them. By law, seniors are not allowed to use their Medicare benefits to pay doctors privately via their own arrangement. Other doctors have not agreed to accept assignment, but they can choose to, on a case-by-case basis. For these "nonparticipating" doctors, Medicare pays 5 percent less than their usual fees. Regardless of how much the health care provider charges non-Medicare patients for the same service, a Medicare patient cannot be charged more than 15 percent over the amount Medicare approves, called the "limiting charge."

By their actions, seniors have shown the path toward Medicare reform—and that path is private insurance. While most beneficiaries continue to select traditional Medicare, that should not necessarily be interpreted as an endorsement of traditional Medicare. Only 23 percent of Medicare users rely solely on that coverage. In fact, more than 70 percent of Medicare beneficiaries already purchase private insurance to supplement or replace traditional Medicare.[5] About 23 percent of beneficiaries buy "Medigap" plans. These state-based private insurance plans that supplement non-drug Medicare benefits are available only to those enrolled in traditional Medicare (A and B) and not to MA enrollees. Twenty-two million beneficiaries, 34 percent, enroll in alternative Medicare Advantage private health plans, with the catastrophic coverage that is missing from traditional Medicare, a total doubling in the past decade.[6] Private prescription drug coverage in Part D, also with catastrophic caps, has also been highly favored and is used by millions of beneficiaries.

President Trump and his administration have made significant strides in improving choice under Medicare since taking office, particularly in the Medicare Advantage part of the program. Nationwide, 3,148 private insurance plans now participate in MA, and the average Medicare beneficiary can choose from twenty-eight plans offered by seven firms in 2020. Nationally, the increase is 15 percent over 2019 and provides the largest number of plans in the history of the program. The continual increase in choices of coverage under MA from nineteen in 2016 to twenty-eight in 2020 reversed the trend of reduced choices under the Obama administration, when thirty-three plans offered in 2010 declined to eighteen in 2015. These private plans provide extra benefits not covered by traditional Medicare. Health and Human Services Secretary Alex Azar announced that average premiums for MA plans will drop by 23 percent compared to 2018—down to the lowest monthly premiums since 2007—likely a result of competition among insurers. This reduction in premiums began in 2016 and reversed the increases seen from 2012 through 2015 under the Obama administration.[7]

Several significant problems exist in these private MA plans. First, Medicare defines minimum required coverage benefits, instead of allowing consumers to use their benefit to choose from cheaper, less-comprehensive levels of coverage. Second, Medicare ultimately defines the actual prices for medical care via complex capitated payments and benchmarks, thereby controlling what care is available.[8] Third, Medicare pays the insurer a fixed amount per enrollee to provide benefits, based on a calculated benchmark cost of coverage. If a plan's bid (premium) is higher than the benchmark, enrollees pay the difference with a monthly premium, in addition to the Medicare Part B premium. If the bid is lower than the benchmark, the plan and Medicare split the difference (called a "rebate")—the patient does not receive this money, other than in part and indirectly, via some form of added benefit coverage that they may or may not want or prefer.

The Goals of Reforms: Simplify Coverage, Improve Choices, and Reduce Costs by Competition

Modernizing Medicare for the twenty-first century is both necessary to save it and an opportunity to improve it as the population ages. The plan centers on a three-pronged strategy that will simplify

Medicare by reducing dependence on fragmented and confusing coverage, add more choices of coverage for seniors, and reduce costs for beneficiaries and all taxpayers. This strategy will empower seniors to choose affordable private health insurance and HSAs, keys to improving benefits and reducing costs by competition for patients. The three elements of the strategy—an incentivized, defined-contribution model, markedly expanded HSAs, and modernization of eligibility—are discussed in detail below.

Element #1: A Defined-Contribution Model

The first element of Medicare reform is implementing a defined-contribution model that offers private insurance options for beneficiaries with competition-based premiums and simplified benefits, as well as consumer incentives to seek value. The basic concept of this model is similar to the Medicare Advantage model: the government would make a defined, fixed contribution, that is, a "premium support," to the private health plan of a Medicare enrollee's choice. There are three significant differences between this new Medicare and current Medicare Advantage. First, new Medicare will make market-based payments to competing insurance plans, rather than setting prices on costs of coverage and then paying health care providers. Second, the required coverage will be determined by beneficiaries' choices, rather than being set by Medicare itself. The array of plans available would be far larger, because the government's role changes from being a direct insurer defining coverage to helping beneficiaries buy insurance they actually want for themselves and their families. Third, if beneficiaries choose a plan with premiums less than the fixed benefit, the "rebate" will go directly to the beneficiary's HSA instead of being seized by Medicare and the insurer. This adds new incentives for beneficiaries to choose coverage with value in mind.

Similar to a number of other reform proposals, the amount of the government's defined-contribution benefit will be based on the average of the three lowest-priced plans put forth to Medicare.

This index group forming the calculated benchmark would include one limited-mandate high-deductible plan. All Medicare-eligible plans would be required to have annual out-of-pocket limits, that is, the catastrophic coverage that is missing from current traditional Medicare.

As noted, if a beneficiary chooses a plan with a premium less than the benchmark, then a rebate payment of the entire difference would be made into that individual's HSA; if payment was due from the enrollee because of costs higher than the benchmark, the enrollee would be responsible. This would save more than the $15 billion per year estimated by the CBO based on using higher benchmarks.[9] In this plan, the taxpayer premium subsidies for the highest income earners would be lower and completely phased out at the highest levels. Medicare enrollees would be able to purchase more coverage by paying more in addition to the fixed government contribution.

Coverage would simplify the current separation of inpatient and outpatient expenses, unifying deductibles and payments fragmented into Medicare Part A and Part B. Ultimately, the goal is to eliminate the confusing and unnecessary separation of all inpatient and outpatient coverage, including for MA plans and prescription drug coverage. In the long run, traditional Medicare will have been moved to private health insurance to improve access to doctors, hospitals, and modern medical technology and drugs; to improve benefits; and to reduce costs for all enrollees. For those over age thirty-five today, traditional Medicare will still remain an option; for those under age thirty-five, traditional Medicare coverage will no longer be provided.

Element #2: Expanded Eligibility and Uses of Health Savings Accounts

The second important element of modernized Medicare is new access to broadly expanded HSAs for all beneficiaries. Presently, HSAs are quite limited in their allowed role for seniors. In fact, as noted earlier, the current laws prohibit HSA eligibility for Medicare enrollees. Seniors who have applied for or accepted Social Security cannot contribute to an HSA. Restricted accounts called Medicare Advantage MSAs are currently available but require enrollment in a high-deductible MA health plan. Among other restrictions (see "Key Questions and Answers on the Atlas Plan"), deposits into these MSAs are prohibited except from Medicare itself and are limited in amount to typically less than half of the required deductible of the accompanying coverage. On the death of the owner, HSAs are deemed taxable unless the beneficiary is the spouse.

Given that future health care needs for today's seniors now last decades, expanded HSAs will be of great importance to a modernized Medicare. HSA holders also participate more in wellness programs that focus on obesity and other major risks associated with chronic disease, increasingly relevant to senior care. New Medicare HSAs will be transformed into highly flexible vehicles for seniors to seek the best value for their health care spending (see "Key Questions and Answers on the Atlas Plan"). Under this plan, Medicare enrollees will automatically receive HSAs if they had none before entering Medicare eligibility. Also under this plan, all Medicare enrollees will be fully eligible for HSAs regardless of enrollment in any specific coverage or program and without any specified level of deductible on insurance. The only requirement for making contributions to the HSA will be that the enrollee have catastrophic coverage. HSAs under new Medicare will have far higher maximum contribution, matching all other HSAs in the newly reformed system limits (see chapter 4); likewise, they will have the same broadened uses of non-Medicare HSAs, including nonprescription medications and home health care devices. All current Medicare MSA limits and rules for use will be updated to match universal HSA regulations, including removing the requirement to enroll in coverage with arbitrarily defined deductibles and eliminating Medicare MSA's restrictions on deposits. Because seniors typically incur greater health care costs, they will be allowed to roll over, tax free, money from retirement accounts into their HSAs. Seniors, their families, and their employers will all be allowed to contribute to the new HSAs up to the annual maximum. People will also be permitted to use their own HSA dollars for the health expenditures of their elderly parents regardless of tax dependency status. Even if Social Security benefits have begun, seniors will still be allowed to fund their HSAs. In new Medicare HSAs, a 20 percent penalty will be in place for nonqualified HSA withdrawals once the owner of the HSA becomes seventy years old. On the death of an enrollee, new Medicare HSA balances will be allowed to be rolled over to the tax-free HSA of the surviving spouse or other family members. This feature will also enhance HSA balances of younger family members and perpetuate increased consumer leverage on pricing.

Element #3: The Modernization of Eligibility

The third element of Medicare reform is the updating of eligibility from obsolete criteria of fifty years ago to reflect the demographics and health needs of today's seniors. The rationale to change these archaic eligibility criteria is straightforward. Modern medical care in the United States has increased life expectancy from birth by 1.6 years per decade for a half century. Life expectancy from age sixty-five has increased about five years since program inception, equating to about one year more from age sixty-five per decade that passes. Thus those individuals currently thirty-five years old will add another three years to their post-sixty-five life span. Moreover, older people now remain in the workforce longer. Retirement age has increased by five years since the early 1990s.[10] Under the proposed new Medicare, the age of eligibility would increase by two months per year until it reaches seventy; after that, the eligibility age would be indexed to life expectancy. From CBO estimates, savings of about $65 billion over the decade would result from slowly phasing in this change.[11]

CHAPTER SIX

Reform #5:
Overhaul Medicaid
and Eliminate the Second-Class
System for Poor Americans

Principal Features of Reform #5: Overhaul Medicaid and Eliminate the Second-Class System for Poor Americans

- Provide private insurance options for all adult Medicaid enrollees without need for special waivers.

  - Permit all insurers, including all companies available on state and federal exchanges, to offer true high-deductible, LMCC plans (covering hospitalizations, outpatient visits, diagnostic tests, prescription drugs, and mental health) to those eligible for Medicaid and the entire state population.
  - Eliminate the requirement of special waivers for Medicaid enrollment into private insurance.

- Establish and seed-fund HSAs for all Medicaid enrollees.

  - Open an HSA automatically for every Medicaid enrollee (*limits and uses to match other HSAs*).
  - Create new incentives for healthy behavior, which will save and protect growing financial assets.
  - Ensure that seed funding goes directly into HSAs as part of federal contribution every year.
  - Permit tax-free rollovers of all HSAs to surviving family members.

- Change the role of Medicaid agencies to assist in managing HSAs and finding private insurance options.

Although it has several different roles and components, Medicaid is generally a subsidy for the poor, paid by federal funds and state funds. Medicaid is intended to help provide access to good medical care and improved health for those who cannot afford it. While the ACA reduced the percentage of uninsured Americans, most of the new coverage came via Medicaid expansion for adults. The CBO estimates that number to grow to 64 million people by 2028. Yet traditional Medicaid is substandard insurance, which most doctors—even half of doctors who signed contracts to accept Medicaid patients—do not even accept (Figure 6.1), according to Department of Health and Human Services (HHS) data.[1] Moreover, the quality of medical care is inferior under Medicaid, according to peer-reviewed medical journals. Lower quality means more in-hospital deaths, more complications from surgery, shorter survival after treatment, and longer hospital stays than similar patients with private insurance.[2] These poor outcomes are most likely due to Medicaid's stricter limits on covered diagnostics, drugs, and treatments, as well as coverage that pays less than the cost of delivering the medical care. Instead of providing a pathway to excellent health care for poor Americans, however, the ACA expansion of Medicaid continued their second-class health care status, and it does so at a cost of $630 billion per year to taxpayers, a cost that will rise to $992 billion in 2027.[3]

As an alternative, a few states had taken the lead within the confines of the ACA via special waivers to facilitate a transition into private coverage with better access to medical care, although implementation has been difficult. Arkansas and Iowa have received approval to use the "private option," in which Medicaid provides premium assistance to purchase private plans in lieu of direct Medicaid coverage.[4] In Arkansas, about 85 percent of Medicaid beneficiaries are now eligible for the private option, and as of January 1, 2015, Iowa has used it as an option for enrollees with income between 100 percent and 133 percent of the federal poverty level. Although these Medicaid pilot projects are still burdened with a

FIGURE 6.1. Percentage of doctors* accepting new Medicaid patients, 2009 versus 2013 overall, in fifteen US major metropolitan areas (*top*); percentage of Medicaid-contracted providers who could offer an appointment to a new Medicaid patient, by type of provider, 2014 (*bottom*).

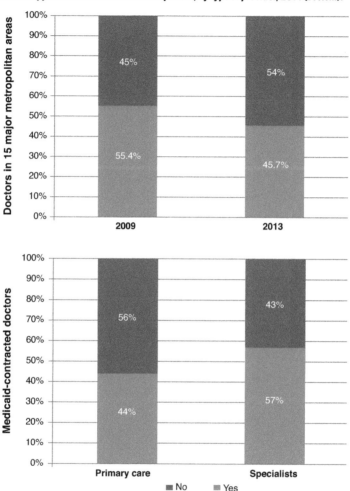

Most doctors do not accept Medicaid patients, and the proportion of doctors who accept new Medicaid patients has been decreasing. Even of the doctors already contracted by Medicaid and listed as accepting patients, a large percentage do not accept new Medicaid patients. Obamacare has massively expanded Medicaid enrollment, but most enrollees will not be able to find doctors who will accept them as patients.

Note: Includes cardiology, dermatology, obstetrics and gynecology, orthopedics, and family practice.

Sources: Merritt Hawkins, *Physician Appointment Wait Times and Medicaid and Medicare Acceptance Rates, 2014 Annual Survey*, http://www.merritthawkins.com/uploadedFiles/MerrittHawkins /Surveys/mha2014waitsurvPDF.pdf 2014 (*top*); Department of Health and Human Services, *Access to Care: Provider Availability in Medicaid Managed Care*, Report OEI-02-13-00670, December 2014, http://oig.hhs.gov/oei/reports/oei-02-13-00670.pdf (*bottom*).

mandated set of benefits and other regulations under the ACA, these states' efforts are steps in the right direction.

The time is long overdue for a fundamental overhaul of Medicaid, with more aggressive reforms to truly modernize it into a program with improved benefits and ultimately reduced costs. Moreover, it seems indefensible to expand a program that is not accepted by most doctors, has worse outcomes than the alternative of private insurance, costs hundreds of billions of dollars per year, and is frankly coverage that none of the members of Congress who expanded it would likely accept for their own families. The goal is to increase access to quality medical care and improve health, not simply label people as "insured."

My plan transforms Medicaid into a bridge program geared toward enrolling beneficiaries into affordable private insurance instead of a parallel second-class system funneling low-income families into substandard traditional Medicaid coverage. The plan establishes and seed-funds HSAs with current funding, a vital component of empowering enrollees with the same control and incentives as all other Americans, while instilling incentives for good health. Note that 60 percent of Medicaid money is spent for outpatient care,[5] and outpatient nonemergency care is amenable to patient choice. HSA reform necessarily goes hand in hand with eliminating anticonsumer regulations that limit competition among doctors and hospitals: this is essential to give empowered patients choices for spending their HSA money. Of particular importance to lower income groups is increasing the available supply of cheaper and more convenient neighborhood primary care. These reforms would change the purpose and culture of Medicaid agency offices from running special government-administered Medicaid plans to establishing HSAs and finding private health plans for Medicaid beneficiaries.

The new Medicaid will have several features. First, new Medicaid will include an LMCC private insurance option for all enrollees, without any need for special waivers. Second, new Medicaid will establish and seed-fund HSAs for the program's low-income

American enrollees, in turn creating growing assets and incentiv-
izing healthy lifestyles to protect those assets. To ensure the availability to Medicaid enrollees of the same health care as is available
to Americans outside the program, federal funding will be available only to states that offer the same private coverage options
to the entire state population, including Medicaid-eligible and
noneligible families. Funds would be allocated via fixed dollar
amounts to states, but directly applied to individual HSAs or
insurance premium payments rather than inefficient state bureau-
cracies. Ultimately, traditional Medicaid coverage will be eliminated over decades as new enrollees move toward private plans
with HSAs.

The new Medicaid will financially empower low-income Americans to (1) purchase affordable private insurance identical to what
any American citizen could buy; and (2) fund HSAs that provide
control and choice and, just as important, build assets worth protecting. These incentive-based Medicaid reforms would move
Medicaid enrollees to private coverage, with equal access to doctors, specialists, treatments, and medical technology. This plan
would eliminate the two-tiered health system furthered by the
ACA Medicaid expansion. It would give control of the health care
dollar to low-income families and foster provider competition for
that money. Medicaid HSAs would provide new incentives for
lower-income families to seek good health through wellness
programs and healthy behavior in order to save and protect their
new, growing financial assets. With these reforms, doctors and
hospitals would receive payments from the same insurance used
by non-Medicaid patients; the limits in access and treatment
options would be eliminated, and costs would come down.

CHAPTER SEVEN

Reform #6:
Strategically Increase Health Care Supply, Create Transparency, and Foster Innovation

Principal Features of Reform #6: Strategically Increase the Supply, Create Transparency, and Foster Innovation

- Facilitate price and value transparency by empowering patients with tools and information, and outlawing obstacles to price visibility.
- Loosen scope-of-practice restraints on nurse practitioners and physician assistants.
- Encourage streamlined training programs for physicians and abolish artificial restrictions on the supply of trained specialists.
- Institute national physician licensing via state reciprocity.
- Minimize obstacles and unnecessary regulatory burdens to stimulate private retail clinics staffed by nurse practitioners and physician assistants for simple primary care.
- Eliminate archaic, anticompetitive state-based certificate-of-need requirements for new technology.
- Streamline the Food and Drug Administration (FDA) processes for device and drug approvals.
- Expose prescription drugs to competition through incentives for patients to seek value and elimination of anticonsumer middlemen and the opaque rebate system.
- Implement strategic immigration reforms to target high-skilled foreign workers and facilitate longer-term visas for highly educated immigrants.

Challenges to high-quality health care access cannot be met without strategically modernizing the supply and delivery of medical care. This became front and center during the recent COVID-19 pandemic, when unprecedented demand for emergency health care supplies, technology, drugs, and personnel stressed our health care system and required on-the-fly mobilization strategies. However, this is not solely an issue for crisis situations. Even after positioning patients with the incentives and authority to choose their own health care and seek value as they define it, the supply of medical care providers and products competing for patients must be increased. Price transparency and understandable indicators of quality are also absolutely essential for value-seeking consumers. In addition to the previously described reforms in this proposal, much of this is accomplished by selective deregulation and eliminating overtly anticonsumer obstacles that preserve a quasi-monopolistic system. The ACA regulatory environment encouraged a record pace of consolidation across the health care sector, including mergers of doctor practices and hospitals to create quasi-monopolies.[1] In the five years leading up to the ACA passage, hospital mergers averaged about fifty-six per year; over the five years since ACA implementation, that number nearly doubled, with 2015's pace the highest in fifteen years. This is bad for patients, because research has generally shown that prices are lower when there are more competing hospitals for insurers to contract with.[2] Insurance premiums are also lower in markets with more hospitals and physicians, as the CBO stated in its 2016 report *Private Health Insurance and Federal Policy.* The last period of hospital mergers increased medical care prices substantially, at times over 20 percent, according to a Robert Wood Johnson Foundation report.[3] Robinson and Miller reported that when hospitals owned doctor groups, per-patient expenditures were 10–20 percent higher, or an extra $1,200–$1,700 per patient per year.[4] Capps, Dranove, and Ody found that physician prices increased on average by 14 percent for medical groups acquired by hospitals; specialist prices increased by 34 percent after joining a health system.[5] In the wake of ACA regulations, overall health care expenditures continued to increase while choices narrowed—for individuals, for employers, as well as for taxpayer-funded government programs.

Increasing the Supply of Medical Care

As the need for medical care explodes, Americans face a shortage of doctors for the entire spectrum of illness. Private-sector clinics owned by pharmacies and staffed by nurse practitioners and physician assistants can provide routine primary care, including administering flu shots, monitoring blood pressure, conducting blood tests, and dispensing inexpensive drugs. In a 2011 review, researchers found that eleven medical conditions (outside of preventive care and immunizations) accounted for 88 percent of acute care visits to retail clinics; all the treatments involved relatively low medical costs.[6] Care initiated at retail clinics is 30 to 40 percent cheaper than similar care at physician offices and about 80 percent cheaper than at emergency departments.[7] Patients seek care at these clinics for several reasons, particularly convenience (that is, extended hours, no need for appointments, and convenient locations), low-cost services, short wait times, and transparent pricing;[8] they have generally reported high levels of satisfaction with their care. Accenture estimates that retail clinics can potentially save hundreds of millions of dollars per year while increasing neighborhood access to routine primary care.[9] While private ownership by stores or pharmacies is common, an emerging trend is for independent retail clinics to develop formal relationships with hospital systems or physician groups. The number of such clinics in the United States exceeds two thousand. Visits to these clinics have nearly doubled over the past five years among commercially insured Blue Cross Blue Shield (BCBS) members,[10] although they are still underutilized. Nearly all accept private insurance (97 percent) and Medicare fee for service (93 percent),[11] but only 60 percent accept traditional Medicaid, the coverage used by the most underserved population, who might benefit the most from lower-cost, more convenient neighborhood clinics.

The key to the proliferation of these clinics rests on eliminating counterproductive obstacles to their use and educating patients about their value. The clinical role of nurse practitioners, many of whom staff such clinics, is governed largely by state scope-of-practice laws that determine the range of services allowed and the extent to which they can practice independently.[12] These laws vary widely and are often unnecessarily restrictive. Starting first with the states categorized as having "restricted practice" regulations, states should revisit outmoded scope-of-practice limits on nurse practitioners and physician assistants.[13] Credentialing requirements for insurance reimbursement should also be simplified.

States should also modernize physician licensing. Nonreciprocal licensing by states unnecessarily limits patient care. To free up capacity for crisis situations, as well as improve access to care in underserved areas, let's replace archaic state-by-state licensing with modern national MD licensing. This will facilitate competition and allow lower-cost telemedicine to grow. Medical school graduation numbers have stagnated for almost forty years, despite widely recognized doctor shortages. It is also time to relax tight limits on physician supply and bring to light the strictly controlled training practices in place for decades. Part of this can be addressed by streamlining training programs.

Increasing physician supply and competition is not only necessary for primary care. Almost two-thirds of the doctor shortage of 124,000 projected for the year 2025 will be in specialists and surgeons, not in primary care (Figure 7.1).[14] In today's health care, virtually all patients with serious diseases are cared for by specialists. For seniors, visits to specialists have increased from 37 percent of visits two decades ago to 55 percent today.[15] That is appropriate, because specialists are the doctors who have the necessary training and expertise to use the complex diagnostics, new procedures, and novel drugs of modern medicine. Patients and policy makers should realize that *despite widely known projections of doctor shortages,* residency and fellowship training programs still find it extraordinarily difficult to increase the number of their trainees, even when

FIGURE 7.1 Projected physician shortages, by field and year, median ranges.

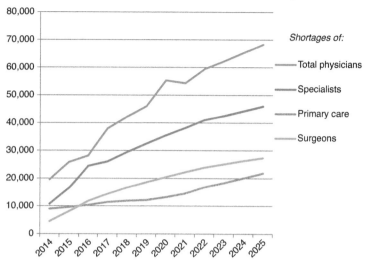

The projected shortages of specialists and surgeons exceed the projected shortage of primary care doctors.

Source: IHS Inc., *The Complexities of Physician Supply and Demand: Projections from 2013 to 2025*, Association of American Medical Colleges, March 2015, doi: DOI: 10.13140/RG.2.2.13111.57764.

fully paying for the additional positions. Professional medical organizations harm consumers by artificially restricting the supply of doctors and lobbying to eliminate competition. These anticonsumer practices need to be opened to public scrutiny or abolished.

We should also eradicate archaic barriers to medical technology and prescription drugs that impede competition and raise prices to patients. Although originally intended to "restrain health care facility costs," the certificate-of-need (CON) requirements are another example of overregulation with unintended consequences, limiting competitive technology in thirty-four states, Puerto Rico, and the District of Columbia.[16] In addition, we need to eliminate excess regulatory barriers that hinder the development of medical technology and drugs. Developing new drugs now takes about fourteen years and costs more than $2.5 billion, a cost that has multiplied tenfold in the past decade.[17] According to a 2010 survey of more than two hundred medical technology companies, delays for approvals of new devices had at that time become far longer than in Europe.[18]

The FDA under the Trump administration has already made progress in facilitating drug approvals: 2017 saw sixty-eight new drugs and biologics approved and a 60 percent increase in generic approvals over the previous year. Over the years 2017 and 2018, average new prescription drug approvals as well as generic approvals increased by approximately 70 percent relative to 2008–16 under the previous administration.

Improving Transparency of Price and Quality

Price transparency is essential for value-seeking consumers using their power to force down prices and improve quality. Instead of following the model of the ACA and single-payer systems, where price is intended to be of no concern to patients, this is central to lowering the price while simultaneously generating high-quality goods and services. These moves are intended to remove the cloak of mystery around health care prices—a harmful situation unique to health care, the only good or service in America that is bought and used without knowing its cost. Yet laws forcing visible prices are not needed for other items. Why not? *Because no one would buy something without knowing its price . . . if they were consciously paying for it themselves.*

And that's precisely the reason why patients don't typically ask about prices. America's health insurance model has evolved to minimize patient out-of-pocket payment. The ACA doubled down on that counterproductive idea. In America today, most doctors and hospitals typically don't bother to compete on price. Note that patients would immediately demand provider prices for most medical care if widespread and reformed HSAs were paired with high-deductible plans. That's because most health care involves smaller, noncatastrophic expenses, and thus far more patients would pay directly for the bulk of their medical care events. That means those prices would naturally align with what consumers value rather than being set artificially or generated via obscure, complex third-party payer arrangements. *Ultimately, the most compelling motivation for doctors and hospitals to post prices and signals of quality would be their understanding that they are suddenly competing for price-conscious patients who control the money.*

The current administration has correctly focused on improving price transparency in its plan to reduce the cost of health care. President Trump signed a legal requirement barring pharmacy gag clauses under Medicare Part D plans, clauses that had prohibited pharmacists from volunteering that a medication may be less expensive than an insurance co-pay if purchased for cash—as was the case more than 20 percent of the time.[19] A separate executive order will require providers paid by Medicare to post prices for a range of procedures. Meanwhile, the Centers for Medicare and Medicaid Services (CMS) recently finalized its mandate requiring pharmaceutical manufacturers to disclose the list price of prescription drugs in direct-to-consumer television advertisements. The Trump administration also announced a proposal to do away with rebates paid by drug manufacturers to pharmacy benefit managers (PBMs), replacing them with discounts to beneficiaries (patients) at the point of sale. PBMs are middlemen that control "formularies," the lists of drugs covered by a plan. Rebates from drug companies to PBMs are payments for influence—either to position a drug on the formulary as "exclusive" or to give it preferred status over competitors. PBMs act counter to patient interests while aggravating the lack of price transparency. These complex behind-the-scenes rebates—$179 billion in 2016—reward inflated list prices, on which patient premiums are often based.[20] This prevents patients from taking account of price.

Price transparency is absolutely critical to lowering the cost of health care, but it alone is not enough to maximize the impact of consumer decision-making on prices. Once empowered patients have strong incentives to seek value from competing providers, they need tools to assess both price and quality. A growing number of tools are now becoming available to compare prices. CMS finalized a rule in 2018 requiring Medicare Part D drug plans to provide electronic tools to doctors that would at least allow discussion with patients regarding out-of-pocket costs for prescription drugs at the time a prescription is written. CMS also updated its guidelines requiring hospitals to post standard medical care charges via an online, patient-friendly platform. Several states have put forth their own laws to require price transparency in health care,[21] and insurers, employers, and even providers increasingly offer price transparency tools.[22] Some physician specialties have recognized the need themselves; for example, several web-based resources have been developed to improve price transparency in oncology.[23] Thorough research demonstrates that consumers will seek lower-priced, high-quality providers when given the right information. However, results to date are mixed, mainly due to two fundamental problems: (1) price transparency from the perspective of providers or policy makers does not necessarily lead to transparency in the type of "price" most relevant to patients—*the out-of-pocket costs*; and (2) today's insurance and other regulations reduce patient motivation to care about price.

High drug prices represent an especially difficult issue. Drugs are the most significant reason for the past half century's unprecedented gains against the deadliest, most debilitating diseases. Here is the long-standing conundrum: the same policies that are associated with the lower prices seen in other countries—price regulation and weaker patent rights—are also associated with delayed launches and reduced access to drugs.[24] Historical evidence shows that facilitating market entry to enhance competition among drug makers is an effective tool to dramatically lower prices (see Figure 7.2A). But we also see an extraordinary lack of price transparency for drugs, fueled by complex behind-the-scenes arrangements with PBMs, as well as insurance that minimizes any possible price consideration by patients. The hidden truth is that prices vary tremendously between drug stores for the same exact drug, yet patients are not sufficiently incentivized to alter buying patterns. According to a December 2017 study, the national average price for a one-month supply of five common generics ranged by a *factor of twenty* between different retailers for a given drug.[25] Even in a single city, the thirty-day supply price showed a *tenfold to seventeen-fold* variation per drug. For the nearly 40 million seniors taking five or more medications daily, the savings from price comparison shopping could be hundreds of dollars per month. To be

FIGURE 7.2A. Average generic price and number of manufacturers after initial entry. Top 25 new generics, 2005.

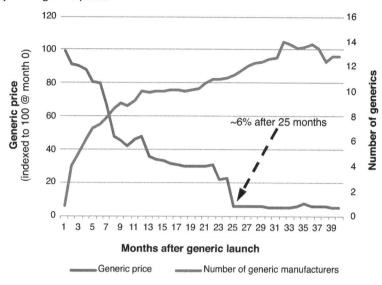

~6% after 25 months

Months after generic launch

Generic price   Number of generic manufacturers

The average generic drug price historically responds to market competition. Prices fall and stabilize to about six percent two years following initial launch, as the number of competing generics enter the market. *Reference:* E. R. Berndt and M. L. Aitken, "Brand Loyalty, Generic Entry and Price Competition in Pharmaceuticals in the Quarter Century after the 1984 Waxman-Hatch Legislation," *International Journal of Economic Business,* 2011; 18:177–201. *Source:* IMS Health, National Sales Perspective, National Prescription Audit: Dec 2009.

most impactful, price transparency must mean visibility of the price relevant to patients—*out-of-pocket costs.* The "retail prices" for my own two prescription drugs are $12.49 and $31.49, but that's not relevant if my out-of-pocket co-payments are less than one dollar each.

Instead of obscuring prices even more with expensive, all-encompassing insurance, changing the model at the pharmacies to increase the frequency of direct payment by patients while rewarding savings via new HSAs would unmask drug prices and instill competition. Many politicians mistakenly push for zero out-of-pocket costs for drugs, but *this is exactly the wrong policy,* as it removes any downward pressure on price from patients, the only end users who personally gain or lose from access to these drugs. I propose cheaper, higher-deductible drug insurance, coupled with large, liberalized-use health savings accounts—a tool especially important for seniors, because they make up about 12 percent of the population but account for over 34 percent of medication use.

FIGURE 7.2B. The inflation-adjusted prescription drug price index has decreased significantly in 2017-19.

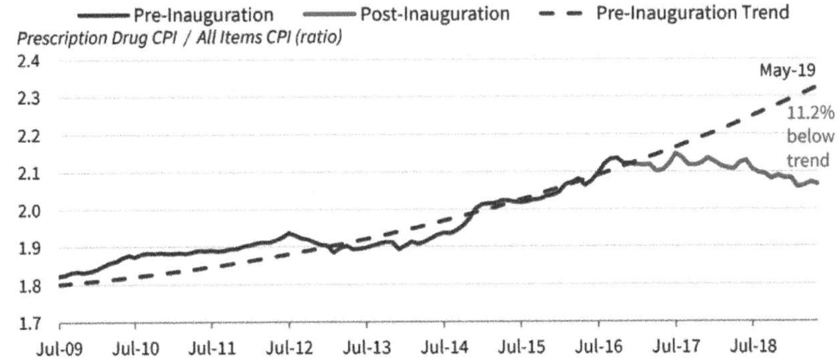

Note: The CPI covers retail transactions, which are about three-fourths of all prescription drug sales. Inflation adjustments are calculated using the ratio of the CPI of prescription drugs relative to the CPI-U for all items. The pre-Inauguration expansion trend in annual growth rates is estimated over a sample period from July 2009 through December 2016, with 2017-18 projected levels then reconstructed from projectead growth rates.
Sources: Bureau of Labor Statistics; Council of Economic Advisers, *Reforming Biopharmaceutical Pricing at Home and Abroad,* February 2018.

That said, the Trump administration has demonstrated that transparency, along with smart deregulation and more competition, can reduce drug prices. As previously noted, during the first two years of the Trump administration, average annual new drug approvals increased by 71.6 percent, relative to the previous eight years under the previous administration. Similarly, average annual generic drug approvals increased by 69.3 percent in 2017 and 2018, relative to 2008–16. *The impact?* The average annual prescription drug inflation (CPI-Rx) was only 2.5 percent, compared with 3.5 percent in 2008–16. That CPI for drugs was also significantly lower relative to the overall inflation index (CPI) during 2017–18 versus during 2008–16 (0.2 percent compared with 1.8 percent). And for the first time in decades, the average price of prescription drugs has declined, from Council of Economic Advisers (CEA) data (Figure 7.2B).

Ensuring Health Care Innovation

Successful innovation depends on many foundational pieces and incentives, including strong intellectual property and patent protection, access to markets, and a host of infrastructural components. Innovation in health care is crucial to advancements against disease, and it is also considered by many to represent the key to reducing costs. Perhaps the most insidious consequence of single-payer health care and the ACA is the threat to innovation—in drugs, devices, and medical technology, the tools that streamline diagnosis, ensure safer treatment, and save lives. The importance of continuing the stream of new drugs, medical technology, and highly specialized, targeted treatments cannot be overstated. We should understand this: the overwhelming majority of the world's health care innovations occur in, and frankly depend on, the United States (Figures 7.3 and 7.4; Table 7.1). These innovations (also see chapter 1 and Figure 1.8) include groundbreaking drug treatments, surgical procedures, medical devices, patents, diagnostics, and much more. For years, the Global Innovation Index report, *R&D Magazine*'s survey of the world's research and development (R&D) leaders, and other publications and indicators have ranked the United States at or near the top for health care innovation, including biopharmaceuticals and medical devices.[26]

But that favorable US environment began to worsen after implementation of the ACA. Growth of total US R&D expenditures from 2012 to 2014 averaged only 2.1 percent, down from an average of 6 percent over the previous fifteen years.[27] Although the slowdown was partly attributable to the weak economy, it was exacerbated by the ACA's new taxes and regulations. According to CBO estimates, the law would have imposed more than $500 billion in new taxes over its first decade, including on manufacturers of medical devices and drugs as well as their investors. Because of that specific tax burden, many small and large US health care technology companies reacted, including Boston Scientific, Stryker, and Cook Medical, all of which announced job cuts and new centers overseas for R&D, manufacturing, and clinical trials.

Health Care as National Security

Concerns about the lack of capacity of medical systems and hospitals to deal with intensive-care unit (ICU) and critical care needs

FIGURE 7.3. First launches of new cancer drugs by country, 1995–2005 (*top*); early availability of new cancer drugs launched 2009–14, by country, as of 2014 (*middle*); US share of first launches of new active substances, world market by year, 1990–2010 (*bottom*). (Also see Figure 1.7.)

First launches of new cancer drugs by country, 1995–2005

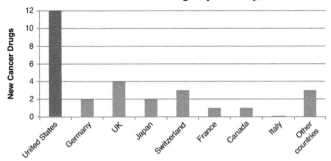

Early availability of new cancer drugs launched 2009–14

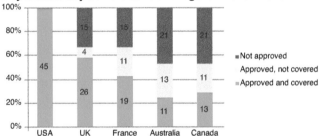

US share of first launches of new active substances, world market, by year, 1990–2010

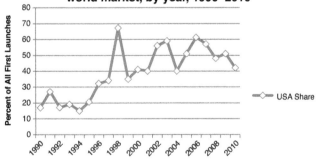

The United States has been the dominant initiator of new drug launches, including new cancer drugs, originating about half of the entire world's new active substances for almost two decades. *Sources:* B. Jonsson and N. Wilking, "Market Uptake of New Oncology Drugs," *Annals of Oncology* 18, suppl. 3 (2007): iii2–iii7, doi: 10.1093/annonc/mdm099 (*top*); Y. Zhang, H. C. Hueser, and I. Hernandez, "Comparing the Approval and Coverage Decisions of New Oncology Drugs in the United States and Other Selected Countries," *Journal of Managed Care and Specialty Pharmacy* 23, no. 2 (February 2017): 247–54 (*middle*); US Food and Drug Administration, *FY 2011 Innovative Drug Approvals*, November 2011, http://www.fda.gov/downloads/AboutFDA/ReportsManualsForms /Reports/UCM278358.pdf (*bottom*).

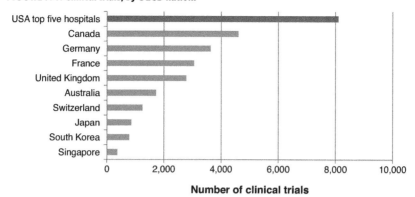

FIGURE 7.4. Clinical trials, by OECD nation.

Number of clinical trials

The top five US hospitals conduct more clinical trials than any OECD nation.
Note: Top five US hospitals as ranked by *US News and World Report*, 2007.
Source: McKinsey Global Institute, *Accounting for the Cost of US Health Care: A New Look at Why Americans Spend More*, December 2008, http://www.mckinsey.com/insights/health_systems_and_services/accounting_for_the_cost_of_us_health_care.

TABLE 7.1. Major medical innovations and country of origin.

Rank	Technology	Description	Country of Origin
1	Magnetic resonance imaging	Noninvasive diagnostic imaging	USA, UK
	Computed tomography		USA, UK
2	Angiotensin-converting enzyme inhibitors	Drugs for hypertension and heart failure	USA
3	Balloon angioplasty	Minimally invasive surgery to unblock arteries	Switzerland
4	Statins	Cholesterol-reducing drugs	USA, Japan
5	Mammography	Breast cancer detection	Indeterminate
6	Coronary artery bypass graft surgery	Surgery for heart failure	USA
7	Proton pump inhibitors	Antiulcer drugs	Sweden, USA
8	Selective serotonin reuptake inhibitors	Antidepressant drugs	USA
9	Cataract extraction and lens implant	Eye surgery	USA
10	Hip replacement	Mechanical prostheses	UK
	Knee replacement		Japan, UK, USA

Source: Based on V. Fuchs and H. Sox, "Physicians' Views of the Relative Importance of 30 Medical Innovations," *Health Affairs* 20 (2001): 30–42.

became a top issue in 2020, as the world grappled with the coronavirus COVID-19 pandemic. No country can realistically have instant availability of unlimited emergency medical care, whether doctors, drugs, or technology. Preparedness can be improved, though, and all systems will now focus on preventing future shortcomings. The COVID-19 pandemic also alerted everyone that health security is a critical part of national security. It provided a moment to re-evaluate and reduce US dependence on other countries, whether allies or adversaries, for critical health needs like pharmaceutical ingredients in advance of the inevitable threats to come, regardless of origin.

The stakes for pharmaceutical supply chains in particular are high even in normal times. Prescription drugs are perhaps the most significant reason for the past half century's unprecedented gains against the deadliest, most debilitating diseases, acute and chronic. More than 15 million seniors in the United States, one of three, take five or more medications daily.[28] And as the US population ages, our society will become even more dependent on drugs. Older people tend to harbor heart disease, cancer, stroke, and dementia—the diseases that depend most on innovative drugs for treatment. Preventing an interruption of the supply of vital medicines that save lives and treat diseases, whether during rare pandemics or in routine medical care, is a matter of national security.

Understanding pharmaceutical supply chains is the first step, and it is not simple. Americans filled 5.8 billion one-month-equivalent prescriptions in 2018,[29] two-thirds of which were for important chronic conditions. That statistic does not include the hundreds of millions of vaccinations on which more than two-thirds of elderly Americans,[30] more than half of America's college students,[31] and more than ninety percent of America's infants and children[32] depend. From 2007 to 2013, imports of drugs and medical devices from China increased nearly fivefold.[33] In 2019, the FDA estimated that about 40 percent of finished drugs and 80 percent of active pharmaceutical ingredients (API), ingredients that produce the intended effect, are manufactured overseas,[34] mainly in China and India. While our pharmaceutical companies have preserved some redundancy in their sources of API for patent-protected brand-name drugs, the generic drug business, accounting for over 90 percent of all prescription medications in the United States, including almost all antibiotics, prioritizes low cost over supply-chain resiliency. Most generics are imported from India, but India receives approximately 70 percent of its APIs from cheaper sources in China. America needs to fully understand and diversify sources of supply, as well as maintain a strategic reserve, of these key drugs.

Beyond the scale and complexity of the supply chain, details on drug manufacturing are opaque. And though the FDA requires country-of-origin markings, the Federal Circuit Court of Appeals ruled in February 2020 that processing ingredients into tablets in the United States is enough to constitute "manufacturing." For instance, a drug manufactured into tablets domestically with API from India may list only the United States as "principal place of business" for FDA purposes.[35] Labeling should be straightforward, but masking important information concerning API origin creates a false sense of security.

Ensuring the supply of prescription drugs also entails protecting against poor quality and counterfeit medicines. The prevalence of impurity, dosing inaccuracy, and overtly fraudulent medication from other countries is difficult to determine precisely, but it poses a significant danger.[36] For instance, a series of fraudulent or contaminated medications have originated in China, including blood pressure medicine[37] and life-saving blood thinners[38] that killed Americans; substandard and fabricated vaccines for children;[39] and fraudulent antibiotics for serious infections shipped all over the world.[40] Simply testing foreign drugs on arrival cannot verify that drugs were manufactured in compliance with US regulations. Although the FDA conducts 3,500 inspections of generic plants a year[41] and requires detailed documentation of compliance, additional measures are necessary to ensure the wholesomeness of imported APIs and drugs. More than half of manufacturing inspections by the FDA are conducted on foreign facilities, but only a small minority are done unannounced in India and China.[42] The US government should require far greater on-site inspection access by the FDA, as well as increase the funding and personnel to implement that policy. It is also time to stop viewing the re-importation of drugs in the pursuit of low prices as without serious downsides, including the risk of interrupted supply and poor quality of many drug imports.[43]

Assessing risk to supply chains should also include an understanding of other countries' dependence on critical US-supplied drugs. The United States is the world's predominant source of pharmaceutical innovation,[44] including development of new cancer drugs, new drugs for rare diseases, "next generation" biopharmaceuticals, and biomarker tests that validate and predict benefit from a given drug treatment. China is highly reliant on foreign sources of more expensive brand-name drugs that make up 90 percent of revenues, exporting only 1.2 percent of all medications by revenue share; the United States is among the top five exporters.[45] China is deeply dependent on US cancer drugs in particular. Of the world's fifty-four new cancer drugs launched from 2013 to 2017,[46] fifty-one (94 percent) were available within two years in the United States while only two were available in China in the same time frame. China's massive problem with cancer[47] is a serious vulnerability, given that its survival rates are only half[48] the survival rates in the United States. That vulnerability is compounded by China's uniquely problematic demographic profile, heavily tilted toward an aging population. In recognition of that vulnerability, China's Healthy China 2030 plan increases the priority of health care, exempts most drugs from taxes,[49] and omits cancer drugs from tariffs placed on other US drugs in 2019. Moreover, China has emphasized the generation of new pharma patents. China's patent applications per year now exceed those from the United States, according to the World International Patent Organization, even though the United States still leads by a wide margin in granted patents.[50] That process will continue to evolve, but mutual dependence on uninterrupted access to critical drugs, among both allies and adversaries, is a vital part of the overall risk mitigation.

What Can Be Done to Support Continued Innovation and Reverse These Damaging Trends?

Congress has already begun part of this restoration by stripping back the ACA's misguided heavy tax burdens on industries and investors, which inhibited innovation, like the ACA's $24 billion medical device excise tax. The Trump administration has also begun to address this by focusing on lower taxes, deregulation, and more transparency, as already noted. The United States needs to retain strong incentives, including specific tax incentives for the high-risk investment crucial to early-stage medical technology and life science companies. It should start by eliminating the higher investment tax instituted as part of the ACA.

Perhaps most important, policies must incentivize pharma innovation and production at home. The key to reducing vulnerability to supply-chain interruption as well as responding rapidly to health threats such as COVID-19 rests on American discovery and competitiveness. The United States leads the world in health care innovation, but the United States should not be complacent. Specific tax incentives for the high-risk investments crucial to early stage medical technology and life science companies are essential to maintaining competitive advantage; incentives could also be introduced for manufacturing critical pharmaceuticals. The FDA must also take a new look at the excessive regulatory barriers that hinder the development of drugs and medical technology while maintaining safety standards at the highest level. Developing new active substances now takes about fourteen years and costs more than $2.5 billion,[51] a cost that has multiplied tenfold in the past decade. Safety standards should not be compromised, but costly, lengthy clinical trials[52] can be streamlined in advance of anticipated infections and other potential threats. The

FDA should also continue the impressive work it began in 2016 to expedite drug approvals.[53] Over the years 2017 and 2018, average yearly new drug approvals increased by approximately 70 percent relative to 2008–16 under the previous administration. Legislators must also avoid the temptation to score short-term political points by imposing price regulation and limiting patent protections. Those policies are harmful, proven to delay drug launches[54] and reduce access to drugs[55] as well as inhibit early-stage R&D projects.[56]

It is also true that Americans pay more for medications than just about anyone else. A 2018 report from the White House's Council of Economic Advisers found that as of 2009, the price per dose of patented drugs was five times as high in the United States as in foreign markets, and US profit margins were four times those in foreign markets.[57] Yet Americans get something important in return (see chapter 1): earliest access to life-saving medications and better treatment results for virtually all serious diseases reliant on drug treatment, including cancer, stroke, heart disease, high blood pressure, and diabetes.

It is critical to avoid policy missteps that have foreseeable but unintended consequences to innovation that ultimately harm patients, especially in drug policy. Many propose price regulation on drugs, but price caps always restrict supply. Cockburn, Lanjouw, and Schankerman showed that price regulation strongly delayed drug launches of 642 new drugs in seventy-six countries.[58] And Santerre and Vernon calculated that drug price controls would have led to 198 fewer new drugs in the US market from 1981 to 2000, at a societal cost of about $100 billion *more than the estimated savings* from those price controls.[59] Pegging our drug prices to those of foreign countries, as proposed by both Senator Bernie Sanders in the Prescription Drug Price Relief Act and the proposed "International Pricing Index" would likely import those price caps and their harms into the United States, even if not circumvented via opaque bundling and other arrangements.[60] This would ultimately lead to the same consequences endured by Europeans in government-dominated systems: reduced access to critical drugs and worse outcomes, including more deaths from disease.

   Price negotiation by Medicare sounds logical, but a single dominant buyer, like Medicare, will lead to supply shortages and fewer new products, as many economists have observed in other industries. But there's a more serious problem ignored by economic analyses. When the negotiator for the buyer isn't the true end user—that is, the patients who use the drugs—only the patient, not the negotiator, will suffer the severe penalties of sickness and death when drug availability and pharmaceutical innovation dry up. The US House of Representatives passed legislation in December 2019 that would allow the federal government to negotiate prescription drug prices with manufacturers as well as impose a 95 percent excise tax on the sales of drugs. From practice, though, we know that "government negotiation" will generate restrictions based on political budgets rather than clinical benefit. *Case in point*: England's NHS launched its new "Budget Impact Test" to delay introducing any new drug for up to three years if projected to exceed £20M in expenditures during any of its first three years, regardless of its cost-effectiveness.[61] NHS patients with cancer, heart disease, and other serious illnesses could be forced to wait years for the "acceptable price" to kick in. One in five new medications were projected to be delayed. Thousands will suffer and die while waiting. By this formula, drugs needed by the largest number of patients would be the very drugs most likely to be delayed. The Alzheimer's Society calculated that a drug costing as little as £23.50 *per year per patient* ($30.26, or under nine cents per day) would still be subject to the new restriction, despite massive societal and individual savings from disease modification. *Would any fully informed American voluntarily transfer such authority over personal health care access to such arbitrary government rules?* It makes more sense to focus on fixing the bloated bureaucracy that has evolved to generate the massive costs and time delays in new drug development.

   Finally, to ensure clinical innovation, we must also keep attracting top students into medicine. Specific estimates vary, but while the direct payments for malpractice amount to less than 1 percent of health spending, if one includes the $45 billion in costs of defensive medicine, the total tallies 2.4 percent of health care spending, or more than $55 billion per year.[62] Therefore, we need to rein in malpractice lawsuits that waste money and discourage pursuit of careers in top, higher-risk specialties. And innovative programs to streamline training and reduce the costs of medical education should be pursued.

Intelligent immigration reform is also important to encourage educated, highly skilled entrepreneurs to stay in the United States. Many of the best and brightest who come to the United States to study science, technology, engineering, and math—subjects crucial to health care innovation—are now choosing to return to their home countries after they finish their studies. In contrast to a decade ago, when from 66 percent to more than 90 percent of foreign students studying in the United States remained here after they completed their studies, only 6 percent of Indian, 10 percent of Chinese, and 15 percent of European students more recently expect to make America their permanent home.[63] Although some of this shift is undoubtedly the result of improving opportunities in those students' home countries and other incentives for them to return home, many graduates want to remain in the United States but are unable to do so. Lawmakers should take a fresh look at easing counterproductive immigration restrictions. New skills-based visa programs should be instituted that specifically target highly educated individuals, particularly students completing American university graduate-degree programs in the areas of science, technology, engineering, and math.

Key Questions and Answers on the Atlas Plan

Reform 1: Expand Affordable Private Insurance

Is there a mandate in the Atlas plan forcing individuals to purchase health insurance?

- No. No one is forced to buy health insurance. It is not the role of the US government to force Americans to purchase a good or service they do not want. That is both anticompetitive and anticonsumer. And the IRS data on the ACA's individual mandate, when it was in place, revealed that 80 percent of households who paid that penalty earned under $50,000 per year—that is, it specifically penalized lower-income people. Moreover, Frean, Gruber, and Sommers stated in the *New England Journal of Medicine* in 2016, "When we assessed the [individual] mandate's detailed provisions . . . we did not find that overall coverage rates responded to these aspects of the law."[1] History has also shown that mandates are typically not very effective and are quite complicated to enforce. The decades of experience in the United States with mandates for automobile insurance and even income taxes show that mandates have a 14 percent to 18 percent noncompliance rate— a percentage strikingly similar to the percentage cited as uninsured before implementation of the ACA, without any mandate.
- My plan takes a different approach: it brings incentives to the system to generate insurance products that are more in line with what consumers want. The plan also gives consumers incentives to buy insurance instead of imposing punishment. This way, consumers will purchase the coverage (and also the health care) that they think is a good value. After all, the money

belongs to the individuals and their families, who earned it, not to the government.

But what about the "free riders" who don't buy insurance? Aren't those of us who buy insurance paying a lot more for our premiums because of them?

■ No. This is one of the great myths behind the idea of forcing everyone to buy insurance. We all care about "fairness," but facts are important. In reality, as Hadley showed in 2008, "private insurance premiums are at most 1.7 percent higher because of the shifting of costs of the uninsured";[2] if a more realistic estimate of cost shifting is used, premiums are less than 1 percent higher due to the shift from people without insurance. This impact is minimal.

Under the Atlas plan, would I be refused care at the emergency room if I had no health insurance?

■ No. My plan does not change the laws protecting uninsured patients. Since the 1986 Emergency Medical Treatment and Active Labor Act, hospitals cannot turn away any individual seeking medical care—regardless of insurance status or ability to pay. Even decades before this law, safeguards for uninsured patients already existed. According to Coughlin et al., $85 billion per year of medical care was administered in 2013 to the uninsured.[3] Roughly $53 billion was paid by federal, state, and local governments. America's doctors contribute another $8 billion per year in free charity care, by various estimates. In 2013, free care was not only given through hospitals; a full 40 percent of free care was given through offices and clinics.

Won't the uninsured people clog up emergency rooms and cause a great financial burden on the rest of us who have insurance?

- No. First, the Oregon study showed that when uninsured people become insured, they use the emergency room more frequently, not less.[4] This finding contradicts the theory that uninsured people overutilize emergency rooms and, with that, shift costs to the insured. Second, the estimated cost shift from the uninsured to insurance premiums paid by the insured is less than 1 percent, a very small amount. This situation will not disappear under my proposal, but it will diminish because (1) more of the poor will have incentives to enroll in coverage (to protect their new assets in HSAs), and (2) the cost of care and insurance will be lower for everyone.

Did the ACA (Obamacare) improve anything about private insurance? If so, does this plan keep those features?

- Yes. Obamacare eliminated lifetime caps on total benefits and prevented insurers from dropping already insured people if they were diagnosed with a disease. Obamacare also put in place annual out-of-pocket maximums. These features would be maintained in this plan.

If everyone used high-deductible insurance, wouldn't that eliminate coverage for preventive care and screening, which would now require out-of-pocket payment?

- No. Nearly all plans, including high-deductible insurance, already cover those visits and procedures—that is, they are not subject to deductibles. My plan does not change this. The real problem is that most patients are not aware of this.

What about office visits to doctors? Are they covered in this plan?

- Yes. Every limited-mandate plan will include three routine office visits per year that are not subject to any deductible. This is unchanged from the catastrophic insurance coverage under Obamacare.

Would the new insurance plans require co-pays?

■ The new plans would be designed by insurers responding to what consumers want to buy, not by my plan or the government, so a variety of arrangements is likely. Consumers would decide what coverage suits their needs, just like consumers decide what food to buy, what sort of clothing and shelter they desire, and what level of safety features they value in a car. Individuals would purchase coverage with the level of co-payments that they personally choose. As with all other goods and services in a free market, the private sector responds to consumer demands by designing products that will sell, and explaining the benefits of those products, to meet the demands of the empowered buyers.

Limited-mandate catastrophic coverage would not cover some aspects of medical care that many people want covered by insurance. How would people pay for that type of care under the Atlas plan?

■ People who want coverage for treatments such as chiropractic care, or acupuncture, or even marriage therapy and massage, that is, any benefits not included in this coverage, are still free to purchase more comprehensive coverage. Just as with other sorts of products, if consumers want to purchase products with added features, the free market is always interested in selling those added features. Plans covering all those benefits will remain available, just like today, but the premiums for those expensive policies will not be tax deductible. Alternatively, people who value that type of service could pay out of pocket from their HSA balances when that service is desired. And prices of all medical care would come down as this competition-based model was implemented.

Aren't you forcing people to buy a specific type of insurance?

▪ No. My plan does not force anyone to buy any insurance; there is no mandate or penalty coercing anyone to buy any form of health coverage. The ACA, by contrast, required more bloated, more expensive coverage. My plan increases choices for consumers, instead of forcing people to buy insurance coverage for services that many people do not want and would never use. Instead of mandates, my proposal provides financial incentives to save money by seeking value, as determined by the consumers. The catastrophic coverage that this reform package encourages and makes widely available is insurance that has already proved to be a good value. Consumers have increasingly moved to purchase this type of insurance when it has been available. In addition, my plan will generate more options for individuals. *This plan will reduce the cost of medical care, consequently lowering the cost of all insurance.* Insurers will respond to the new environment where there are fewer restrictions on insurance plans and where consumers are free to look for insurance tailored to their personal goals for coverage. Insurance will cost less under this plan.

Under the Atlas plan, could I be dropped from my insurance if I get a serious disease?

▪ No. Americans who stay in continuous insurance coverage would not be penalized for developing costly diseases. In my plan, you cannot be dropped from coverage if you acquire or harbor a disease once insured; this feature serves as another incentive to become insured and then maintain insured status.

But could I buy insurance in the Atlas plan if I already have a disease, and I did not have insurance beforehand?

▪ Yes, but it would probably cost you significantly more money than if you had bought it beforehand. Obamacare required "guaranteed issue" of insurance. Obamacare prohibited insurers in the individual market from denying coverage, increasing premiums, or restricting benefits because of any preexisting condition. Those rules are actually bad for consumers. First, those rules provided an incentive to those who simply avoided paying for insurance until they acquired a serious disease. This is unfair to everyone else, especially those who took personal responsibility and bought insurance while they were healthy in anticipation of possibly needing insurance to protect against the financial risk of becoming ill. Further, we knew from states' experience with "guaranteed issue" that two things happen: coverage becomes less available because carriers leave the market, and premiums increase for everyone else. States with those regulations are typically those with the least affordable health insurance. The young and healthy—typically those who earn the least and are most likely to be uninsured—are forced to subsidize the rates of older and often wealthier individuals, which also interferes with risk pools. Under Obamacare, new "guaranteed issue" rules increased insurance premiums by about 20–45 percent, according to the Milliman report.[5] My plan is fairer for everyone and better for consumers. It rewards people for being responsible and maintaining insurance, and they cannot be dropped once they become ill.

- In my plan, states will form high-risk pools using new models to help those with diseases buy more affordable insurance. For instance, as a condition for selling insurance in a given state market, private health insurance companies would establish a risk-pooling cooperative into which they would pay premiums to protect against the risk of very high health claims. Premiums would be related to the actuarial value of the risk characteristics of their enrollee populations. Even more important, my plan would lower the cost of insurance for everyone, so more people would be able to afford health insurance before they became ill in the first place.

Under the Atlas plan, will I lose my Obamacare subsidy to purchase private insurance on Obamacare exchanges?

- Yes, but the $850 billion of Obamacare subsidies given to help pay for private insurance under the ACA was harmful, because it propped up insurance and medical care prices by providing insurance coverage for more and more people, which shielded patients from caring about the price of care. Those subsidies were also an example of an irrational use of taxpayer money, because the ACA itself *caused* prices of private insurance to skyrocket. My plan is more sensible: I remove many of the factors (for example, excessive mandates and misguided regulations) that caused the cost of coverage to become so expensive. And my plan reduces the cost of health care itself—the main factor determining insurance premiums. *Under my plan, insurance coverage will become far less expensive,* so people will be able to afford the insurance and actually choose to buy it because it represents a good value. In addition, take-home wages will increase because of the tax reforms in my plan, so Americans will have more money to spend how they choose.

Aren't high-deductible plans just "pseudo-insurance"? It's really not insurance at all, is it?

- That is absolutely wrong. It is a gross misconception that high-deductible coverage is inadequate; for some people, it is exactly what they prefer. The role of insurance is to cover unanticipated large expenses. Assisting people with insufficient means to pay for expected, routine expenses is an entirely separate issue. Homeowners insurance doesn't pay for replacing light bulbs and mowing the lawn. Moreover, it is a harmful policy to bloat coverage with mandates that cause high premiums for everyone, when many people would never choose to pay for that coverage if allowed to choose less-comprehensive plans. *Why would everyone be required to pay for such things as marriage counseling, massage therapy, in vitro fertilization, and chiropractors—examples of the thousands of state mandates—if they know they would never use those services?* Unfortunately, the ACA furthered a misconception about health coverage, and it hurt consumers. ACA regulations caused premiums for high-deductible plans to rise from two to five times faster than premium increases of any other type of coverage. Those regulations need to be removed.

Won't I lose my employer-provided health benefit if the income exclusion is capped that low?

- No. Under my plan, the maximum allowable health benefit provided by employers will be set to match the maximum allowed for an HSA under my plan. That benefit is fully deductible for the employer and the employee under my plan. In addition, economists generally agree that the employer-employee market trades benefits for wages, which implies that competition would force employers to raise wages commensurate with reduced benefits. Employees would receive higher take-home pay.

Shouldn't we eliminate the model of employer-sponsored health benefits?

- No. Employer-paid health benefits and insurance are perhaps the best working model of US health insurance—that's not the problem. As more companies compete for employees, benefits will undoubtedly become even better. The fact that employers are increasingly offering higher-deductible coverage and HSAs as options for their employees is good, because employees should be allowed to decide how to spend their own money on their own health care and health care coverage, and higher-deductible coverage positions patients as the direct buyer. It is true that people should not lose their HSAs if they change jobs or become unemployed, and my plan ensures that.

Won't the Atlas plan, with its removal of certain tax subsidies and other changes, result in millions of people becoming uninsured?

- No. *More people will be insured, because insurance will be less expensive, and medical care will cost less, under my plan.* The prices of health care will decrease as competition ensues and as the counterproductive, perverse incentives in our current system are removed. In my plan, the idea is to generate insurance options that people value and therefore decide to purchase, rather than force people under threat of penalty to buy insurance products that they would not choose to spend their money on. The reforms in this plan will markedly increase the consumer's purchasing power for medical care, and this increase will more than compensate for the loss of tax subsidies for purchasing health care or insurance. Remember, in 2018 under the ACA, 45 percent of uninsured adults said that they remained uninsured because the cost of coverage was too high. This plan will reduce the price of all health insurance, and it will also increase options for lower-cost coverage.

What about prescription drugs, especially for people with chronic diseases? How will they pay for their medications?

- All limited-mandate plans will also include coverage for prescription drugs. And people will still have the same options to buy coverage that includes lower deductibles or even exempts drugs from being subject to deductibles. My plan will result in more choices of insurance coverage, not less, including plans that are cheaper because they have higher deductibles for drugs. That is what experience shows in all other goods or services in a free market: the private sector ultimately supplies products (like different types of insurance coverage) that consumers want to buy; consumers have the control of the money in my plan. Even today, some states already include plans with separate deductibles for prescription drugs; my plan will result in even more of these tailored deductibles. And these new types of coverage for prescription drugs and other reforms described will lower the prices of prescription drugs for patients.

Why doesn't this plan place price caps on prescription drugs?

■ Price caps ultimately do not work to provide the desired products at lower prices. In fact, price caps consistently reduce the supply of the product—this is Econ 101. In this case, that would do great harm to patients, because the number of drugs would become less available. Similarly, pegging our drug prices to those of foreign countries, as proposed by members of Congress, would essentially import their price caps and ultimately their restrictions on availability into the United States, as well as threaten new drug development. My reforms would reduce the cost of drugs by virtue of the following: unleashing the power of consumers through control of payments; ridding our system of the regulatory excesses that generate the massive costs and time involved in new drug discovery; streamlining the overly long approval process for lower-cost generic drugs; eliminating the punitive taxes on the pharmaceutical industry, which are passed on to consumers; and reversing the Obamacare elements that have contributed to ongoing consolidation, which further harms consumers. The biggest danger for Americans, particularly senior citizens, who commonly depend on prescription drugs, is increasing insurer consolidation and government control over decisions on insurance reimbursement. As proved by history and by those countries with government-centralized health care, more government domination over health care results in less access to the life-saving drugs that government bureaucrats judge to be costly or "unnecessary." For example, we see this in such systems as the National Health Service in England and in Canada, with their scandalous waiting lists, limitations on innovative drugs and tests, and worse outcomes than here in the United States.

Why allow insurers to charge higher premiums for obesity? Isn't that discrimination?

■ Just like cigarette smoking, obesity is a high-risk, voluntary lifestyle for most individuals and a major driver of health expense with well-known health hazards. As is the case for virtually every other form of insurance, rates for health insurance that reflect higher risk of disease and more frequent use of medical care as a consequence of voluntary behavior are totally appropriate. For instance, risky driving is a key factor in determining automobile insurance rates. My plan does not discriminate against people who are obese or who smoke; in fact, it extends more help to those who need it, with more wellness programs, including blood pressure and cholesterol screening, nutritional counseling, and exercise training.

Reform 2: Establish and Liberalize Universal Health Savings Accounts

The Atlas plan eliminates the requirement for a government-defined deductible in order to open an HSA. Is any health insurance required to fund the HSA? If so, what type?

■ Yes. To be eligible to contribute to an HSA in any given year, you must also have insurance that covers catastrophic care. My plan does not specify the level of deductible, though; the only contingency is that catastrophic care is covered, whether in a comprehensive plan or not.

But isn't the purpose of the HSA to cover the high deductible, so that health expenses that are smaller than the deductible are paid by the HSA?

■ That's only partly true. Money in an HSA could also be used for co-pays, for example, but not for insurance premiums. The new limits on contributions to HSAs would roughly equal the maximum allowed for annual out-of-pocket spending, including deductibles and co-pays (and those maximums would increase as indexed to the consumer price index). But it might also be valuable to have money in the HSA to pay for medical services that are not covered by the new insurance plan. Remember, many people will probably buy a limited-mandate plan, because it would be cheaper and those people may not want coverage for services they would never use. At some point, an enrollee might want to use an uncovered medical service; that could be paid out of the HSA. And finally, take-home wages will be higher because employers will shift much of the previous payments for tax-preferred benefits to direct wages because of the tax reforms under this plan.

How specifically are the new HSAs liberalized beyond just size?

■ First, expenditures from new HSAs would be permitted not only for the account holder but also for spouses, children, elderly parents, and siblings—regardless of tax dependency on the named account holder. Current law permits expenses only for the account holder, spouse, and tax-dependent children. Second, reformed HSAs will have an expanded list of qualified medical expenses, to include certain over-the-counter drugs and home health care devices. Current law limits HSA expenditures to prescription drugs and insulin. Reformed HSAs will retain tax-sheltered status when passed on to any surviving family member—not just spouses, as is true today. HSAs should be usable for direct primary care payment and other innovative health care payment strategies and coverage that will arise once reforms are enacted to put patients in control of payment.

Why wouldn't people just withdraw money from HSAs for other uses?

- The financial penalty for withdrawals of funds from HSAs for noneligible spending will be significant—in my plan, the penalty will be raised to 50 percent from the current 20 percent.

Do you get to keep the HSA as a tax-sheltered account even if you drop the insurance plan after you have established and funded the HSA?

- Yes. This is the law today, and this plan does not change it.

Would seniors be allowed to withdraw from their HSAs for other reasons outside of health care without penalty?

- Once they reach age seventy, seniors would be allowed to withdraw from their HSAs without the full 50 percent penalty. Nevertheless, the HSA is not intended to be a retirement account for expenditures other than health care. In new Medicare HSAs, a 20 percent penalty would be in place for withdrawals unrelated to health care, starting once the owner of the HSA reaches seventy. And these accounts will now be able to be passed on to living family members without penalty.

People can't really shop for medical care. It's too complicated, isn't it?

- No, it is not too complicated for most individuals. As long as the information necessary to make informed decisions is visible, then shopping for nonemergency medical care would be simple. We know that Americans find it straightforward to shop for computers and other far more complicated items. Under my plan, price transparency and competition create even more visible information for consumers. And remember, most medical care episodes are not an emergency, where life-and-death decisions must be made quickly. The bulk of medical care is scheduled, and most health care involves smaller, noncatastrophic expenses, and that care is amenable to price and quality comparisons.

Why do we need to significantly increase the size of HSAs? After all, with today's limits, most people do not maximize their contributions.

■ Remember, today's high price of medical care and the regulatory burden of Obamacare, which forces the purchase of mandate-filled, expensive insurance, have left the consumer with far less money for funding HSAs. Meanwhile, ACA subsidies for insurance that minimizes out-of-pocket payments have prevented consumers from caring much about medical care prices and have consequently shielded doctors from competing on price. Unpressured prices for medical care plus Obamacare's regulatory burden equals markedly higher insurance premiums (doubled from 2013 to 2017, even with significantly higher deductibles)—and that means less money for HSA contributions. And even with today's counterproductive limitations and insurance regulations, which have dramatically limited the potential benefits of HSAs, and therefore their value, the number of accounts has increased. *By increasingly choosing HSAs when given the opportunity, American consumers are approving their value.*

■ The fundamental impact of HSAs is to reduce the price of health care for everyone, rich or poor, whether or not they have an HSA. With larger and improved HSAs, patients become sensitive to price because they are rewarded by saving money. Widespread large HSAs, when paired with cheaper, high-deductible plans, could pay for the bulk of medical care events. The more people are positioned to pay directly for most of their care, the more downward pressure on prices will occur through providers competing for cost-conscious patients.

If everyone had a new HSA at birth, who would keep track of those accounts?

■ The federal government would be the repository of the information. This is already true—the federal government regulates and keeps track of all HSAs today.

Reform 3: Instill Rational Tax Treatment of Health Spending with Appropriate Incentives

Why not allow income tax exclusions or deductions for all insurance, including low-deductible insurance, if the premiums are low (that is, why not just cap the level of the deduction)?

- The purpose of my tax reform is not solely to limit the amount of the deduction (or income exclusion) in order to remove the harmful incentive to spend more on health care. I also want to remove a tax preference for insurance that hides the costs of that care from patients. It would be counterproductive to allow any tax preference—whether a deduction, an income exclusion, or an HSA expense—for "comprehensive" insurance, because low-deductible, heavily mandated plans hide the costs of covered care. That insurance model is a fundamental cause of lack of access and rising costs for everyone. I want to put the consideration of value and price back into the consumer's purchasing decisions, just as value and price are considered in every other good and service. My plan reforms health insurance back to the way it was intended to function, that is, to cover only *significant* and unexpected costs. That way, individuals are positioned to drive down prices using their power—because they pay directly (up to the deductible), they shop for value, and market forces reduce costs of care down to what consumers determine would be a good value for their money. If people want to buy insurance that minimizes out-of-pocket payment, that's fine, but it should not be incentivized and subsidized by other taxpayers.

What level of deductible does the Atlas plan use to define an insurance plan as "high deductible"?

- My definition of "high deductible" is based on 75 percent of the maximum allowable HSA contribution. For example, to qualify as a high-deductible plan that has tax preference for 2020, during which the allowable HSA contribution will be $8,150, the deductible would be $6,112.50. This linkage would be one way to ensure that the HSA contribution maximum will always be higher than covering just the deductible. But HSA eligibility extends to all plans, regardless of deductible size, because we want to maximize the number of HSAs to maximize downward pressure on the price of medical care and on insurance premiums—and those lower prices impact everyone, even people without HSAs.

Why is the specific amount of $8,150 chosen for the maximum tax exclusion?

- Although like all such thresholds, the selection of such a number is somewhat inexact and arguable, this number was chosen for a few reasons: (1) it matches the 2020 allowed annual out-of-pocket expenses for group health plans under the ACA; (2) it matches the proposed maximum for deductible HSA annual contribution; and (3) it is close to the average annual employer-based health benefit.

Why not allow a tax deduction for all health care spending, instead of limiting the tax preference to HSAs and high-deductible insurance premiums?

- Tax deductions for all health care spending give an incentive to spend more money on health care; in other words, there is an opportunity cost if you spend money on something other than health care because the money is worth more when spent on health care. Why is that sensible, while spending on other essentials, like food and clothing, is not deductible? That preference generates more and more spending on health care rather than on other desired goods and services. My plan eliminates that misincentive. Instead, the incentive is to put money into an HSA and then seek value when it is spent on necessary care; the opportunity cost is when it is spent because it could be saved and then grow by investment (or be bequeathed to the account owner's survivors). Of course, everyone could still choose to spend their own money on nondeductible health care products and services; being nondeductible, consumers would be more concerned with price and value, and prices would come down.

Won't the tax preference for basic catastrophic coverage cause higher prices for that coverage because of subsequent increased demand?

■ Generally, high demand for goods does lead to price increases. However, increasing demand for the insurance itself is not a major driver of the cost of insurance premiums. Health insurance premiums rise mainly in response to increases in the cost of providing health care services, not demand for the insurance itself. Prior and anticipated payouts for medical services are by far the single largest component of health insurance premiums. When the cost of health care services increases, insurance premiums rise. Other factors do have some impact on private insurance premiums, including government regulations, in particular mandated coverage; characteristics of the insured individual (for example, age and certain behaviors); and cost shifting caused by underpayment by public insurance. We need to recognize that the main reason for the lower premiums of catastrophic coverage with high deductibles and fewer mandates lies in the very structure of limited-mandate coverage. Premiums of high-deductible catastrophic coverage are lower than premiums of so-called comprehensive coverage because of the anticipated lower costs of covering the medical care under the plan. In addition, this plan will generate more insurers competing for buyers, another factor proven to generate lower insurance premiums.

Won't the new tax reforms hurt the middle class?

■ No. My tax reforms specifically help the middle class and remove today's tax benefits for more affluent individuals. The *current* tax preference is unfair—it gives a high-value tax deduction for high spending on health insurance that covers everything without limits. This feature overwhelmingly benefits the upper-income earners, that is, the people who enjoy the biggest value from the present tax deduction. The existing tax preference gives a disproportionate benefit to the wealthy because of their higher marginal tax bracket. My plan simplifies the tax reform and removes the special benefit that high-income earners accrue from the current tax exclusion. Ultimately, this plan will reduce the cost of insurance premiums and medical care more than the tax benefit for health spending, which has distorted the market for health care.

- The ACA instituted a new "Cadillac tax"—a 40 percent tax on expensive health insurance plans, and that tax has been repeatedly delayed by Congress. But the logic for that tax approaches absurdity. Obamacare assessed a new tax on health insurance that exceeds a certain price. Obamacare by its own regulations simultaneously caused the prices of health insurance to rise. Therefore, the government ends up imposing a tax on insurance whose price became high, and consequently subject to the tax, directly because of the government's own policy. In addition, the Cadillac tax will count HSA contributions (from employers and individuals) toward the threshold for invoking the tax penalty, thereby penalizing consumers for trying to keep health care costs low.

- My tax plan is simpler and also fairer to everyone, because it levels the playing field. Under my plan, small business employees, part-time workers, and self-employed people will all have the same deduction as those working for large employers. My plan also gives a tax deduction for significantly expanded HSA contributions, which will increase everyone's savings for out-of-pocket medical costs. Moreover, this plan will help the middle class with more affordable insurance coverage and more control of costs because they have new purchasing power.

Won't the new tax reforms hurt employees by reducing benefits because employers will lose some of their deductions for health benefits?

- No. The truth is that to a large extent employees pay for their benefits by receiving lower wages than they would have otherwise been paid. Employment benefits, including health care benefits, replace wages. If I limit the tax deduction for health benefits paid by employers, then employers would likely pay less of those benefits at first. But over time, employees will instead receive higher wages and more take-home pay as employers are forced to compete with higher wages to attract labor.

Won't reducing the allowable income exclusion from taxation constitute a new tax increase and therefore reduce wages?

- No. This six-point health reform plan will reduce the medical care costs by more than the lost value of the old tax exclusion for health benefits to consumers. The proposed tax reform herein is a cut in a tax expenditure program.[6] In addition, the reforms in this plan will increase take-home wages as employer behavior changes in response to the health reform plan.

Reform 4: Modernize Medicare for the Twenty-First Century

Isn't this plan going to destroy Medicare?

- No. Quite the opposite—it's going to save it. My plan will introduce competition among insurance companies, so cheaper insurance options will become available for consumers. This plan will expand choices for beneficiaries, so beneficiaries can decide whether they want more comprehensive coverage or lower-cost insurance coverage. It also helps seniors allocate more savings to cover out-of-pocket expenses through new eligibility for expanded HSAs, and it allows seniors more flexibility on paying for those health-related items from their HSAs. This plan will significantly reduce the cost of Medicare so that it will be available for generations to come. And this long-term viability is crucial because Medicare will be even more important in the future, as more people live longer and medical advances continue. In the long run, traditional Medicare will be moved to private health insurance to improve benefits, reduce costs, and eliminate the increasing problem for seniors of finding doctors and hospitals who accept Medicare. For those over age thirty-five today, though, traditional Medicare will still be an option when they become Medicare eligible.

How is this Medicare reform different from previous reform proposals?

■ This plan shares some key principles of reform with prior proposals, most notably the fundamental idea of defined benefits for premium support and competition among insurers for enrollees. Still, this plan differs from previous proposals in a number of important ways, including the following:

  ● The benchmark used to calculate Medicare premiums would be determined by an average of the three lowest-priced private plans submitted; included in those would be a limited-mandate plan.
  ● New Medicare would contain a major expansion and liberalization of HSAs, including new eligibility for universal HSA ownership and continuing contributions for all beneficiaries; significant expansion of HSA limits; broader HSA uses; new rules allowing transfers from retirement accounts; and new permission to pass on HSA balances to surviving family members.
  ● While everyone over age thirty-five today will still have the option of traditional Medicare, eventually traditional Medi-

care coverage would be phased out entirely so that ultimately all Medicare beneficiaries would have the advantages of private insurance, with better access to doctors, hospitals, drug treatments, and advanced medical technology.

- Instead of sharing rebates with the government after choosing cheaper insurance (as happens today with Medicare Advantage), new Medicare beneficiaries would receive 100 percent of the rebates, in cash returns to their HSAs, if they selected insurance with lower premiums than the benchmark.

- The plan would eliminate the current anticonsumer conflict-of-interest of the federal government that allows government restrictions on access to medical care. Today, with its role as the insurer via traditional Medicare, the government has the power to restrict access to care and artificially set prices for medical services. This ability has already caused a reduction in doctor acceptance of Medicare, and trends show further reductions. Under my plan, traditional Medicare is eventually eliminated, so the government will support beneficiaries with money to buy insurance instead of dictating benefits and prices as an insurer. In the new Medicare, the government will stay out of the way of impeding consumer choice and access to care. With the new plan, the Medicare patient will have the power to choose from the same wide array and state-of-the-art excellence of medical care as everyone else.

How will the Atlas reforms of Medicare deal with risk pools and adverse selection, where some insurers will mainly enroll low-risk, healthier seniors and create far more expensive insurance for those with chronic diseases?

- A risk pool is the basic foundation of health insurance, so that enrollees with lower health care costs offset enrollees with higher health care costs in a large group of enrollees in a given health plan. It is used to spread risk among groups of people enrolled in health plans to allow insurers to manage their ability to pay claims and provide benefits. Insurance markets could be destabilized by a phenomenon called "adverse selection," where sicker individuals enroll in certain plans in a disproportionate number. This causes higher premiums, which in turn cause younger, healthier people to leave the plan, creating a cycle ultimately leading to collapse. Risk pooling is necessary to prevent such spirals. One possible risk pool mechanism would be a risk-adjustment program similar to those proposed by both the Wyden-Ryan plan and the Heritage Foundation's proposal. Participating insurers would be required to establish a national risk pool in order to sell to Medicare beneficiaries. Insurers with higher shares of low-cost enrollees would contribute to a fund that would make payments to insurers with larger shares of high-cost enrollees. Medicare administrators would monitor the enrollment data of participating health plans and require cross subsidies to compensate for plans with a disproportionate enrollment of high-risk beneficiaries. I believe the actual premium changes and calculations of cross subsidies should be performed by the insurers themselves, rather than the government.

How will the coverage of new Medicare insurance plans be determined?

- The coverage and benefits of the new insurance plans will ultimately be determined by the individuals selecting the plans, that is, the Medicare beneficiaries themselves. Under the new Medicare plan, the beneficiaries will have far more choices at competitive prices. Today, overly bloated requirements for coverage that many beneficiaries do not want are causing excessively high premiums and out-of-pocket costs, including the coverage requirements of traditional Medicare. Because beneficiaries would receive rebates in their HSAs if they chose cheaper insurance, they would now have incentives to consider carefully what coverage they chose. Remember, enrollees still have the choice of buying insurance with more extensive coverage. Equally important, as a result of the new competition in place, insurance and medical care itself would cost less under the new reforms to the health care system.

Won't seniors be at greater risk if the government is not the insurer? Who will protect seniors?

■ My plan ensures that seniors will be protected the same way they are now—by the existing Center for Drug and Health Plan Choice, a federal oversight agency that resides within the Centers for Medicare and Medicaid Services. This center would have authority to approve insurance plans that meet standards, just like it does today for Medicare Advantage plans and drug benefit plans competing in today's Part D (nonetheless, it would not have authority to standardize benefits or determine rates). Moreover, the state-based regulatory agencies that currently enforce rules for health insurance and consumer protection against fraud and misleading advertising will also remain in place. This reform plan does nothing to expose seniors to more risk or danger.

What about low-income seniors?

■ Just like today, America's safety net for low-income senior citizens would remain in place for the so-called dual eligible. Medicaid assistance would add to their federal Medicare subsidies. The difference is that under the reforms to both Medicaid and Medicare in this proposal, the choices, the access, and the quality of health care for low-income seniors would be strengthened and expanded.

Will I lose my current doctor whom I have seen for years under Medicare? Seniors have complicated medical problems, so it is very important to have continuity of care.

- No. In fact, my plan will reduce the problem of finding doctors that has already begun. Today, more and more doctors are refusing to see Medicare patients. Traditional Medicare pays doctors less than the cost of providing medical care. In my plan, more Medicare patients will be allowed to buy private insurance identical to that offered to non-Medicare patients, that is, coverage that pays doctors appropriate amounts for care. The plan eliminates the main reason for doctors refusing to accept more patients on government insurance, including Medicare. And the same applies to hospitals. Under this plan, the best hospitals and specialists, the doctors whom seniors need most, will no longer drop Medicare acceptance. Remember, bills proposing Medicare for All immediately reduce payments to providers by approximately 40 percent. . . . Does anyone honestly believe access to timely, high-quality health care and choice of the same doctors and hospitals would not be markedly reduced in that system?

How would beneficiary income be used to determine new Medicare benefits under the Atlas plan?

- My plan is similar to current income adjustments in today's Medicare Part B and Part D, but with some differences. Today, adjusted gross incomes over $85,000 for individuals and $170,000 for joint filers result in higher monthly premiums up to a certain point, with no complete phase-out of taxpayer subsidies. Under my plan, the same phase-in of premium adjustments would occur (subsidies from taxpayers would decrease for those with incomes above these thresholds), but in addition I propose that the highest-income earners (those with adjusted gross incomes greater than $1,000,000 for individuals) receive no subsidies at all.

Will there be a cap on annual out-of-pocket expenses in the new Medicare insurance plans?

- Yes. The maximum allowable out-of-pocket annual expenses for seniors will be matched to the maximum allowable contribution to HSAs. For 2020, that cap will equal $8,150 for self-only coverage and $16,300 for self-and-family coverage, including the deductible. Nevertheless, lower out-of-pocket maximums will likely also be available among the many choices of insurance plans open to seniors in the new Medicare program.

Under the Atlas plan for Medicare, would seniors be at risk of losing coverage for preexisting conditions, and would the "oldest old" of Medicare beneficiaries pay far higher rates?

- No. Nothing would change from the current status of community rating (where premiums would be based on the pool of enrollees, not the individual) and guaranteed issue (where existing health problems would not prevent the individual from obtaining insurance) in the current Medicare program.

What would happen to the complicated rules by which some doctors accept Medicare assignment and others do not?

- Those rules would be abolished. Under this new plan, Medicare beneficiaries would be allowed to purchase medical care with cash, insurance, or any other means of payment agreeable to them and their doctors. And health care providers could accept any means of payment without the current restrictions that interfere with doctor access for Medicare beneficiaries.

How quickly would the age of eligibility for Medicare increase?

- Two months per year—so it would take six years for the eligibility age to have increased by one year, twelve years for it to have increased by two years, and so forth. And it would only affect those currently age fifty or younger. For example, under the current system, people currently age fifty become eligible for

Medicare in fifteen years (in the year 2030). Under my plan, the age of eligibility would increase by thirty months after fifteen years from the implementation of the rule change; therefore, individuals now age fifty would become eligible for Medicare at age 67.5. In 2045, that is, in thirty years, the age of eligibility would be seventy. Any subsequent changes in eligibility age would be related to the increases in US life expectancy.

Will prescription drugs and cancer screening be covered in the new Medicare plans accepted for competitive bidding?

■ Yes. All Medicare insurance plans will include prescription drug coverage, including limited-mandate catastrophic plans. But consumers will have choices as to the deductibles and co-payments, and as with every other good or service, the sellers (insurers) will provide products (insurance) in response to what buyers (patients) demand for their money. As they do today, plans will likely require co-pays, although more choices of coverage and benefits will be available to beneficiaries. All plans will cover the most important cancer screening tests for no out-of-pocket charges, regardless of the deductible.

Isn't this plan just like replacing Medicare with Medicare Advantage (MA)?

■ No. In MA, Medicare defines minimum required coverage, instead of allowing beneficiaries to choose from cheaper, tailored coverage they may desire. Second, in MA, Medicare defines the actual prices for medical care, thereby controlling what care is available. Third, in MA, if a plan's premium is higher than the benchmark, beneficiaries pay the difference, in addition to the Medicare Part B premium. If the premium is lower than the benchmark, the plan and Medicare split the difference (the "rebate"); the patient does not receive this money. In my plan, patients receive the rebate directly into their own HSAs.

Given that seniors have much larger health care usage and costs than other age groups, aren't HSAs going to be too small to have any practical value?

■ No. Under my plan, seniors will have a special allowance to transfer funds from any tax-sheltered retirement account into their HSA without any tax penalty and reversible up to the amount of the transfer. This feature will allow at least some seniors who need a backstop and choose to do so to leverage their new purchasing power for medical care. In addition, seniors who choose coverage that costs less than the benchmark average will receive a rebate into their HSA, that is, money to be used for health care expenses. Lastly, children or other family members will be able to use their HSAs to help pay HSA-eligible expenses. And don't forget that health care itself will cost significantly less.

How do HSA rules under the Atlas Medicare plan differ from current HSA rules for Medicare beneficiaries?

■ Under today's Medicare, HSAs are restricted in several ways, many of which are highly complicated and indeed arcane.

- Current HSAs and Medicare:
  - To qualify for an HSA, you cannot be enrolled in Medicare.
  - Beginning with the first month you enroll in Medicare Part A or Part B, you can no longer contribute any money to an HSA (though you may still withdraw money for eligible expenditures).
  - If you apply for or accept Social Security benefits, even if you continue working, you cannot contribute to an HSA (because once you accept Social Security benefits, you are automatically enrolled into Medicare Parts A and B). Note that you may decline Medicare Part B if you continue to work for a large employer, but you cannot decline Medicare Part A. Also note that you must stop contributing to

your existing HSA six months before you apply for Social Security, or you will owe a tax penalty because Medicare Part A is retroactive for six months prior to the Social Security application.

♦ If your spouse is the designated beneficiary, the HSA will be treated as the spouse's HSA at your death; if not, the account stops being an HSA, and its balance becomes taxable to the beneficiary or the estate.

● Current Medicare Advantage MSAs (tax-exempt Archer medical savings accounts set up with a financial institution into which the Medicare program can deposit money for qualified medical expenses):

♦ These accounts are uncommon and offered on a state-by-state basis.

♦ Eligibility requires Medicare enrollment *and* enrollment in a high-deductible Medicare Advantage health plan that meets Medicare guidelines.

♦ Unlike HSAs, which allow deposits from anyone (yourself, your employer, or other family members), neither you nor your employer is allowed to deposit any money into Medicare MSAs. Only Medicare can deposit money into your MSA.

♦ The deposits into Medicare MSAs are generally significantly less than the deductible of the accompanying high-deductible plan, typically less than half.

♦ In general, you cannot have other health insurance that would cover the cost of services during your Medicare MSA plan's yearly deductible.

♦ Many people are ineligible for a Medicare MSA, including those who have health coverage that would cover the Medicare MSA plan deductible (including benefits from an employer or union group health plan), Medicaid enrollees, and those who relocate outside the service area of the plan.

- ◆ If you withdraw money for nonqualified expenses, the money becomes taxable, and a 50 percent penalty is charged regardless of the age of the beneficiary.
- ◆ If you name a beneficiary for your MSA account who is not your spouse, the money in the account after your death becomes taxable and is added to that person's income when he or she files that year's income tax return.

■ Under my new Medicare proposal, the following rules would be in place:

- All Medicare enrollees are eligible for new Medicare HSAs regardless of enrollment in any or all Medicare coverage.
- No specific deductible is required on an accompanying insurance plan to contribute to a new Medicare HSA. The only requirement for contributing is having catastrophic coverage, regardless of the level of deductible.
- Instead of the confusing, complex allowance for HSA spending by those over age sixty-five on certain insurance premiums (that is, they can reimburse themselves for the money that Social Security withholds to pay Medicare Part B and can make tax-free HSA withdrawals to pay Medicare Part D and Medicare Advantage premiums but not Medigap premiums), new HSAs will permit tax-free spending for all premiums of all high-deductible plans.
- New Medicare HSA contribution limits are significantly higher than current HSA limits and current Medicare MSA limits, and they match all other non-Medicare HSA limits.
- New Medicare HSA uses are broadened to match all other non-Medicare HSA uses, including, for example, nonprescription medication.
- New Medicare HSA contributions are open to employers, family members, and individuals.
- New Medicare HSA contributions are allowed even for individuals receiving Social Security benefits.

- Once they reach age seventy, seniors would be allowed to withdraw from their HSAs without the full 50 percent penalty. In new Medicare HSAs, a 20 percent penalty would be in place for withdrawals not used for health care once the owner of the HSA reached seventy.
- On the death of the senior, new Medicare HSA balances could be bequeathed to the tax-free HSA of a surviving spouse or family members.

Isn't the Atlas plan really just "privatization" of Medicare into a voucher plan?

- Regarding privatization, this plan preserves the federal government benefit of health insurance for senior citizens, with both taxpayer money and administrative oversight by the government. Remember, the reality of current Medicare is that about 70 percent of beneficiaries already supplement or fully replace traditional Medicare with private insurance. Only about 13 percent of beneficiaries have traditional Medicare alone. The private insurance offered in this new Medicare will have numerous advantages for beneficiaries over current insurance options, as described elsewhere in this book. Remember also that the best access to care and the best outcomes from care come from private insurance, not government insurance. This has been proved both here in the United States (for example, the Veterans Health Administration system or Medicaid) and around the globe, where patients in government-centralized systems experience unconscionable waits for care and worse outcomes than care obtained via private insurance. Do not forget another fact: the private insurance of current Medicare Advantage plans outscored traditional Medicare on nine of eleven measures of health care quality in a recent direct comparison[7] and as reviewed in the *New England Journal of Medicine* by Guram and Moffit.[8] The bottom line is that this reform plan removes government from an inherent conflict of interest—being not only the insurer but also the dominant insurer, with direct or indirect control over nearly all prices and access to care. This fundamental change will increase the availability and quality of medical care and reduce its cost for seniors.

■ Regarding vouchers, no, this is not a voucher plan. In a voucher system, a set amount of money (typically indexed in some way to something that changes over time, such as the consumer price index) is sent to the beneficiary. Then, the beneficiary is basically on his or her own to use it in the purchase of private coverage. My proposal involves premium support, whereby Medicare would pay a certain amount (determined by the Medicare benchmark calculation rather than indexed to anything other than the market price for private insurance by way of competing plans submitted for bid) to a Medicare-approved health plan. In this proposal, seniors are not fending for themselves with vouchers.

Under the Atlas plan, if a beneficiary selects coverage with premiums that are lower than the new Medicare benchmark payment, the beneficiary would receive a rebate. Is that the same as the rebate offered today under Medicare Advantage?

■ Not exactly. The proposed plan is more advantageous for consumers. Under current Medicare Advantage, if the selected plan is less than the government's benchmark payment, the plan by law returns 75 percent of the savings to the beneficiary by way of more benefits, and the remaining 25 percent goes to the government. In my plan, the entire savings—100 percent—goes directly to the consumer in cash, as a deposit to the consumer's HSA; the government receives nothing.

Reform 5: Overhaul Medicaid and Eliminate the Second-Class
System for Poor Americans

How will the poor get started with HSAs to get into the Atlas health care plan?

- All individuals, including all Medicaid beneficiaries, will own HSAs. Under this plan, Medicaid agencies would assist in educating enrollees about managing HSAs, as well as in finding and enrolling them in private plans.

Would current holders of traditional Medicaid suddenly lose their insurance?

- No. They would have the new option of switching to new Medicaid (private high-deductible insurance with money going into their own HSA immediately); in this plan, over a period of ten to twenty years, I envision that traditional Medicaid will be gradually phased out for most Medicaid holders through their own choices. Ultimately, Medicaid will then have been fully transformed into a private insurance premium support program.

Why would doctors suddenly accept new Medicaid patients when they do not accept them now?

- In traditional Medicaid, the payments for medical services are very low, even below cost in many cases. Under the new plan, doctors and hospitals would receive payments from the same private insurance (or HSAs) as with any other non-Medicaid patient; doctors and hospitals would not even know who was a Medicaid patient and who was not. This plan allows Medicaid patients to receive care from the same doctors and hospitals that everyone else uses.

What new incentives for healthy lifestyles and preventive care would exist under new Medicaid?

■ New Medicaid patients would have the same doctors as private patients. Medicaid patients would receive counsel and the offer of the same screening tests and wellness information as all privately insured patients. In addition, new Medicaid enrollees would have new assets to protect as their HSA balances are built up. The existence of these new assets would provide an incentive for long-term protection. Remember, the rationale for insurance is to cover possible loss of assets; this is also one of the main motivators for receiving preventive care and living a healthy lifestyle.

Reform 6: Strategically Increase Health Care Supply, Create Transparency, and Foster Innovation

Is it realistic to propose streamlined training programs for physicians?

■ Yes. Innovative, shortened training programs already exist. For example, the NYU School of Medicine has begun offering a streamlined three-year medical degree program. The Texas Tech University School of Medicine and others are also offering accelerated programs.

Why not just pass laws requiring price transparency?

■ First, price transparency is essential, but it is not sufficient. And second, we may not need specific legislation to force price transparency. Indeed, laws forcing visible prices are not needed for other items. Why not? *Because no one would buy something without knowing its price . . . if they were consciously paying for it themselves.* Uniquely in health care, government regulations themselves have undermined price visibility, by pushing people toward insurance that minimizes out-of-pocket payments so that patients perceive that "someone else is paying." Along with misguided tax incentives, regulations have prevented consumers from caring about medical care prices. My overall plan is intended to remove the cloak of mystery around health care prices. First, patients must directly gain from paying less. Second, patients must pay directly for more of their own care. To position patients as direct payers for a higher proportion of their medical care, cheaper, higher-deductible insurance plans with larger, more valuable HSAs must become available to everyone rather than being limited. Although not necessarily appropriate for everyone, when given the opportunity, patients increasingly opt for lower-cost, higher-deductible insurance, and these plans put patients directly in position to pay for care. Transparency requirements instituted by the Trump administration have definitely shown some positive results, but direct payment by patients with strong personal incentive to seek value is the most powerful lever for reducing costs of care while improving quality.

Why would you call for loosening immigration limits? Don't immigrants take jobs from American citizens and cost taxpayers money through our public schools and our entitlement programs?

■ The immigration reforms suggested in this plan specifically target highly educated, entrepreneurial immigrants who would be here legally. These people are extremely important contributors to American innovation and job creation in our society—they come to the United States for education and opportunity, not for entitlements. Moreover, foreign-born people are more likely than US-born people to start a company, according to Fairlie's 2012 study.[9] And according to the Kauffman Foundation, about 44 percent of engineering and technology companies founded between 2006 and 2012 had at least one founder who was born abroad.[10] Our health care system would benefit, by way of important advances, new jobs, and more tax revenues, from the efforts of highly educated people.

What is the total cost of the Atlas health plan?

■ My plan will reduce national health expenditures, and consumers will save on insurance and health care. Nonetheless, it is difficult at best to separate and project over the long term the extremely complex and overlapping impacts of health system reforms. Moreover, in the context of cheaper medical care that will clearly result from these reforms, I have not included any of the other positive economic impacts, such as the anticipated rise in employee wages or job growth as a consequence of the reforms outlined in this plan. Given those limitations, I estimate the financial impacts from this plan over the first decade using reasonable approximations based on published literature and previous estimates of the JCT and the CBO, as indicated in Tables Q&A.1 and Q&A.2.

TABLE Q&A.1. Impact of Atlas plan on private savings and costs, over decade (approximations).

Specific Reform	Estimated Savings (Loss) over Decade (in $billions)	Reform Category (See Plan)
Remove penalties on uninsured people and employers	$210*	Reform #1: Private insurance expansion
Remove excise tax on health insurance premiums	$87*	Reform #1: Private insurance expansion
Premiums from shift to lower-cost, limited-mandate coverage[1]	$940†	Reform #1: Private insurance expansion
Expanded HSA enrollment and limits[2]	$350†	Reform #2: Universal liberalized HSAs
Transparency to consumers[3]	$880†	Reform #2: Universal liberalized HSAs
Expanded utilization of wellness and lifestyle programs[4]	$120†	Reform #2: Universal liberalized HSAs
Reduced income exclusion	($550*)	Reform #3: Tax reforms
High-deductible option and new, expanded HSAs[5]	$400†	Reform #4: Medicare modernization

(continued on next page)

TABLE Q&A.1. (continued)

Specific Reform	Estimated Savings (Loss) over Decade (in $billions)	Reform Category (See Plan)
Gradually phased-in increase in age of eligibility	($64*)	Reform #4: Medicare modernization
High-deductible option and new, expanded HSAs[6]	$50†	Reform #5: Medicaid overhaul
Repeal of taxes on devices and brand-name drugs	$196*	Reform #6: Supply increases
Increased supply of retail clinics[7]	$20†	Reform #6: Supply increases
Medical liability reforms[8]	$110†	Reform #6: Supply increases

Overall Net Private Savings‡
$2,749,000,000,000 (~$2.75T), over decade

[1] Estimated 5 percent savings per year from current projections on total private premiums paid, based on half of the 63 percent of privately insured who were not already in high-deductible plans switching, estimated 10 percent overall price drop in high-deductible plans from reduced mandates and more competition among insurers, and estimated 10 percent lower premiums for all existing and future high-deductible health plans extrapolating from one-half of other competition-induced health care price decreases. Data from US Department of Health/CDC/National Center for Health Statistics, June 2015 (see Table 10 in *Health Insurance Coverage: Early Release of Estimates from the National Health Interview Survey*, 2014); and CMS (see Exhibit 2 in S.P. Keehan et al., "National Health Expenditure Projections, 2014–24: Spending Growth Faster Than Recent Trends," *Health Affairs* 34(8) (2015): 1407–17, http://content.healthaffairs.org/content/early/2015/07/15/hlthaff.2015.0600).

[2] Estimated from extrapolating extra savings from HSAs on expenditures with high-deductible plans of 5.5 percent to 14.1 percent (see A.M. Haviland et al., "The Effects of Consumer-Directed Health Plans on Episodes of Health Care," *Forum for Health Economics and Policy* 14(2) (2011): 1–27, http://www.rand.org/pubs/external_publications/EP201100208.html); overall estimate of 5 percent expected additional savings in all health expenditures for non-senior citizens because of widespread HSA enrollment.

[3] Estimated from transparency impact on reductions in spending for outpatient services assuming 19 percent reduction. See S. Wu et al., "Price Transparency for MRIs Increased Use of Less Costly Providers and Triggered Provider Competition," *Health Affairs* 33(8) (2014): 1391–98, http://content.healthaffairs.org/33/8/1391.abstract; and J.C. Robinson, T. Brown, and C. Whaley, "Reference-Based Benefit Design Changes Consumers' Choices and Employers' Payments for Ambulatory Surgery," *Health Affairs* 34(3) (2015): 415–22, http://content.healthaffairs.org/content/34/3/415.abstract); projected outpatient spending in employer-sponsored insurance (see Haviland, 2011, cited above, and A.M. Haviland et al., "Growth of Consumer-Directed Health Plans to One-Half of All Employer-Sponsored Insurance Could Save $57 Billion Annually," *Health Affairs* 31(5) (2012): 1009–15, http://content.healthaffairs.org/content/31/5/1009.full.

[4] Estimated from impact of multiple wellness programs on health spending, based on $200/year/employee savings and 50 percent employee participation. See American Institute for Preventive Medicine, *Health and Economic Implications of Worksite Wellness Programs*, 2010; also Bureau of Labor Statistics.

[5] Estimated for new money into HSAs, reduced payments of premiums for supplemental insurance, rebates to enrollees choosing low-premium plans, and savings for out-of-pocket Medicare health expenses.

[6] Estimated for new money into HSAs and accumulated savings resulting from consumer incentives and high-deductible plans for nondisabled, non-senior adult enrollees into Medicaid.

[7] Estimated from J. Spetz et al., "Scope-of-Practice Laws for Nurse Practitioners Limit Cost Savings That Can Be Achieved in Retail Clinics," *Health Affairs* 32(11) (2013): 1977–84.

[8] Estimated to save 20 percent of total annual associated costs of medical liability. See M.M. Mello et al., "National Costs of the Medical Liability System," *Health Affairs* 29(9) (2010): 1569–77.

*Approximations based on CBO/JCT estimates over one decade of implementation.

†Other amounts derived from the literature, using conservative estimates and given expected price transparency and increase in higher deductibles with HSAs.

‡Not including anticipated rise in wages to employees resulting from response to health reforms.

TABLE Q&A.2. Impact of Atlas plan on government spending, over decade (approximations).

Specific Reform	Estimated Spending Reduction over Decade (in $billions)	Reform Category (See Plan)
Eliminate ACA exchange subsidies	$822*	Reform #1: Private insurance expansion
Premium support with competitive bidding	$275*	Reform #4: Medicare modernization
Fixed federal grants to states, capped by CPI-U annual increases	$450*	Reform #5: Medicaid overhaul

Overall government spending reduction:
$1,547,000,000,000 (~$1.5T) less, over decade

*Approximations based on CBO/JCT estimates over one decade of implementation.

Notes

Chapter 1

1. Organisation for Economic Co-operation and Development, 2018 Data on Health Spending, https://data.oecd.org/healthres/health-spending.htm.

2. US Census Bureau, "The Next Four Decades: The Older Population in the United States: 2010 to 2050 (Based on 2008 Data)," https://www.census.gov /prod/2010pubs/p25-1138.pdf.

3. F. Islami et al., "Proportion and Number of Cancer Cases and Deaths Attributable to Potentially Modifiable Risk Factors in the United States," *CA: A Journal for Clinicians* 68, no. 1 (2018), doi: 10.3322/caac.21440.

4. Organisation for Economic Co-operation and Development, *OECD Fact Book 2018* (Paris: OECD, 2018).

5. A. M. Sisko et al., "National Health Expenditure Projections, 2018–27: Economic and Demographic Trends Drive Spending and Enrollment Growth," *Health Affairs* 38 (2019): 491.

6. "Estimated Medicaid and CHIP Enrollment Data," August 2019, Medicaid .gov; R Rudowitz, E, Hinton, and L, Antonisse, "Medicaid Enrollment & Spending Growth: FY 2018 & 2019," Kaiser Family Foundation.

7. Centers for Medicare and Medicaid Services, *2019 Annual Report of the Boards of the Federal Hospital Insurance and Federal Supplementary Medical Insurance Trust Funds*, April 2019.

8. National Research Council and National Academy of Public Administration, *Choosing the Nation's Fiscal Future* (Washington DC: National Academy of Sciences, 2011).

9. World Health Organization, *The World Health Report 2000: Health Systems: Improving Performance* (Geneva: WHO, 2000).

10. See C. Almeida et al., "Methodological Concerns and Recommendations on Policy Consequences of the *World Health Report 2000*," *Lancet* 357 (2001): 1692; Y. Asada and T. Hedemann, "A Problem with the Individual Approach in the WHO Inequality Measurement," *International Journal for Equity In Health* 1 (2002): 2; P. Musgrove, "Judging Health Systems: Reflections on WHO's Methods," *Lancet* 361 (2003): 1817–20; V. Navarro, "Assessment of the World Health Report 2000," *Lancet* 356 (2000): 1598; E. Ollila and M. Koivusalo, "The *World Health Report 2000*: The World Health Organization Health Policy

Steering Off-Course: Changed Values, Poor Evidence, and Lack of Accountability," *International Journal of Health Services* 32 (2002): 503–14; C. J. L. Murray et al., *Overall Health System Achievement for 191 Countries*, Global Program on Evidence for Health Policy Discussion Paper Series no. 28 (Geneva: WHO, n.d.), 8, fig. 1.

11. "Ill-Conceived Ranking Makes for Unhealthy Debate," *Wall Street Journal*, October 21, 2009.

12. R. Woods, "Long-Term Trends in Fetal Mortality: Implications for Developing Countries," *Bulletin of the World Health Organization* 86 (2008): 417.

13. W. C. Graafmans et al., "Comparability of Published Perinatal Mortality Rates in Western Europe: The Quantitative Impact of Differences in Gestational Age and Birthweight Criteria," *British Journal of* Obstetrics *and* Gynaecology 108 (2001): 1237.

14. M. F. MacDorman and T. J. Mathews, "Behind International Rankings of Infant Mortality: How the United States Compares with Europe," *International Journal of Health Services* 40 (2010): 577.

15. World Health Organization, *Neonatal and Perinatal Mortality: Country, Regional and Global Estimates* (Geneva: WHO, 2006), https://apps.who.int/iris/handle/10665/43444.

16. M. Heron, "Deaths: Leading Causes for 2016," *National Vital Statistics Reports* 67, no. 6 (2018).

17. J. O'Neill and D. M. O'Neill, "Health Status, Health Care and Inequality: Canada vs. the U.S." NBER Working Paper 13429, National Bureau of Economic Research, September 2007; D. M. Cutler, A. Garber, and D. P. Goldman, eds., *Frontiers in Health Policy Research* 10 (2007).

18. A. Baer and P. E. Graves, "Predicting Life Expectancy: A Cross-Country Empirical Analysis," University of Colorado, 2002, https://spot.colorado.edu/~gravesp/WPLifeExpectancy6-6-02.htm.

19. Global BMI Mortality Collaboration, "Body-Mass Index and All-Cause Mortality: Individual-Participant-Data Meta-Analysis of 239 Prospective Studies in Four Continents," *Lancet* 388 (2016): 776.

20. B. Forey, J. Hamling, P. Lee, and N. Wald, *International Smoking Statistics: A Collection of Historical Data from Thirty Economically Developed Countries* (Oxford: Oxford University Press, 2002).

21. National Center for Health Statistics, Health, United States, 2014; Table 15. Life expectancy at birth and at age 65, by sex: Organisation for Economic Cooperation and Development (OECD) countries, selected years 1980–2012.

22. M. Palacios and B. Barua, "The Price of Public Health Care Insurance, 2019," *Fraser Research Bulletin*, Fraser Institute, August 2019.

23. B. Barua and S. Hasan, "The Private Cost of Public Queues for Medically Necessary Care, 2018," Fraser Institute, https://www.fraserinstitute.org/studies/private-cost-of-public-queues-for-medically-necessary-care-2018.

24. C. Blahous, "The Costs of a National Single-Payer Healthcare System," Mercatus Center, George Mason University, Government Spending Working Papers, July 30, 2018.

25. For a detailed review of the literature, see S. W. Atlas, *In Excellent Health* (Stanford, CA: Hoover Institution Press, 2011), 159–209.

26. B. Barua, *Waiting Your Turn: Wait Times for Health Care in Canada*, Fraser Institute, 2017, https://www.fraserinstitute.org/studies/waiting-your -turn-wait-times-for-health-care-in-canada-2017.

27. R. J. Blendon et al., "Confronting Competing Demands to Improve Quality: A Five-Country Hospital Survey; Amid Common Concerns about Quality, Hospital Leaders Endorse Investing in Information Technology," *Health Affairs* 23 (2004): 119, doi: 10.1377/hlthaff.23.3.119.

28. J. Z. Ayanian and T. J. Quinn, "Quality of Care for Coronary Heart Disease in Two Countries," *Health Affairs* 20 (2001): 55–67.

29. Merritt Hawkins, *2009 Survey of Physician Appointment Wait Times*; Merritt Hawkins, *2017 Survey of Physician Appointment Wait Times*, September 2017, https://www.merritthawkins.com/news-and-insights/thought-leadership /survey/survey-of-physician-appointment-wait-times; Merritt Hawkins, "Physician Appointment Wait Times and Medicaid and Medicare Acceptance Rates, 2014 Annual Survey," http://www.merritthawkins.com/uploadedFiles/Merritt Hawkins/Surveys/mha2014waitsurvPDF.pdf.

30. B. Barua, N. Esmail, and T. Jackson, *The Effect of Wait Times on Mortality in Canada*, Fraser Institute, 2014.

31. V. Stevanovic and R. Fujisawa, "Performance of Systems of Cancer Care in OECD Countries: Exploration of the Relation between Resources, Process Quality, Governance, and Survival in Patients with Breast, Cervical, Colorectal, and Lung Cancers," HCQI Expert Group meeting, Paris, 27 May 2011.

32. B. Jonsson and N. Wilking, "Market Uptake of New Oncology Drugs," *Annals of Oncology* 18(suppl. 3) (2007): iii2–iii7, doi: 10.1093/annonc/mdm099.

33. S. A. Roberts, J. D. Allen, and E. V. Sigal, "Despite Criticism of the FDA Review Process, New Cancer Drugs Reach Patients Sooner in the United States Than in Europe," *Health Affairs* 30 (2011), https://doi.org/10.1377/hlthaff.2011.0231.

34. US FDA Center of Drug Evaluation and Research, *Novel Drugs 2015 Summary*, January 2016.

35. C. Troskie et al., "Regulatory Approval Time for Hormonal Contraception in Canada, the United States and the United Kingdom, 2000–2015: A Retrospective Data Analysis," CMAJ Open 2016.

36. Y. Zhang, H. Hueser, and I. Hernandez, "Comparing the Approval and Coverage Decisions of New Oncology Drugs in the United States and Other Selected Countries," *Journal of Managed Care and Specialty Pharmacy* 23 (2017): 247–54.

37. IQVIA Institute, *Global Oncology Trends 2019: Therapeutics, Clinical Development and Health System Implications*, 2019, data via *Statista*,

https://www.statista.com/statistics/696020/availability-of-new-oncology-drugs
-by-country.

38. NHS England, "Changes to NICE Drug Appraisals: What You Need to Know," National Institute for Health and Care Excellence (NICE), April 4, 2017, https://www.nice.org.uk/news/feature/changes-to-nice-drug-appraisals-what -you-need-to-know.

39. D. H. Howard et al., "Cancer Screening and Age in the United States and Europe," *Health Affairs* 28 (2009): 1838–47.

40. O'Neill and O'Neill, "Health Status"; Cutler, Garber, and Goldman, *Frontiers.*

41. For a detailed review of the literature, see Atlas, *In Excellent Health*, 97–157.

42. A. Verdecchia et al., "Recent Cancer Survival in Europe: A 2000–02 Period Analysis of EUROCARE-4 Data," *Lancet Oncology* 8 (2007): 784–96; Concord Working Group, "Cancer Survival in Five Continents: A Worldwide Population-Based Study," *Lancet Oncology* 9 (2008): 730–56.

43. P. Kaul et al., "Long-Term Mortality of Patients with Acute Myocardial Infarction in the United States and Canada," *Circulation* 110 (2004): 1754–60.

44. See, for example, F. Levi et al., "Trends in Mortality from Cardiovascular and Cerebrovascular Diseases in Europe and Other Areas of the World, *Heart* 88 (2002): 119–24; P. Kaul et al., "Long-Term Mortality"; M. L. Martinson et al., "Health across the Life Span in the United States and England," *American Journal of Epidemiology*, March 9, 2011, doi: 10.1093/aje/kwq325; J. Z. Ayanian and T. J. Quinn, "Quality of Care for Coronary Heart Disease in Two Countries," *Health Affairs* 20 (2001): 55–67; H. C. Wijeysundera et al., "Association of Temporal Trends in Risk Factors and Treatment Uptake with Coronary Heart Disease Mortality, 1994–2005," *Journal of the American Medical Association* 303 (2010): 1841–47; K. E. Thorpe, D. H. Howard, and K. Galactionova, "Differences in Disease Prevalence as a Source of the US-European Health Care Spending Gap," *Health Affairs* 26(suppl. 2) (2007).

45. Outpatient hypertension treatment, treatment intensification, and control in Western Europe and the United States. Y. R. Wang et al., "Outpatient Hypertension Treatment, Treatment Intensification, and Control in Western Europe and the United States," *Archives of Internal Medicine* 167 (2007): 141–47.

46. See, for example, K. Wolf-Maier et al., "Hypertension Treatment and Control in Five European Countries, Canada, and the United States," *Hypertension* 43 (2004): 10–17; Y. R. Wang et al., "Outpatient Hypertension Treatment; E. Gakidou et al., "Management of Diabetes and Associated Cardiovascular Risk Factors in Seven Countries: A Comparison of Data from National Health Examination Surveys," *Bulletin of the World Health Organization* 89 (2011): 172–83.

47. S. Neville, "NHS Funds Diverted to Private Sector," *Financial Times*, March 26, 2017.

48. K. Socha and M. Bech, "Extended Free Choice of Hospital—Waiting Time," *Health Policy Monitor*, October 2007, http://www.hpm.org/survey/dk/a10/1.

49. C. Blahous, "Single-Payer."

50. GAO Highlights 15-448, *Medicare Program: Additional Actions Needed to Improve Eligibility Verification of Providers and Suppliers*, June 2015.

51. Office of the Inspector General, Report No. A-09-16-02023, February 2018.

52. J. Cubanski et al., "Sources of Supplemental Coverage Among Medicare Beneficiaries in 2016," Kaiser Family Foundation, November 2018 Data Note.

53. J. Gruber and K. Simon, "Crowd-Out Ten Years Later: Have Recent Public Insurance Expansions Crowded Out Private Health Insurance?" *Journal of Health Economics* 27 (2008): 201–17.

54. W. Fox and J. Pickering, "Hospital and Physician Cost Shift: Payment Level Comparison of Medicare, Medicaid, and Commercial Payers," Milliman Client Report, December 2008, http://www.milliman.com/expertise/health care/publications/rr/pdfs/hospital-physician-cost-shift-RR12-01-08.pdf.

Chapter 2

1. Centers for Studying Health System Change, "CTS Physician Surveys and the HSC 2008 Health Tracking Physician Survey," http://www.hschange.com/index.cgi?data=04.

2. Merritt Hawkins, *2017 Survey*.

3. Department of Health and Human Services, "Access to Care: Provider Availability in Medicaid Managed Care," Report OEI-02-13-00670, December 2014, http://oig.hhs.gov/oei/reports/oei-02-13-00670.pdf.

4. K. Holgash and M. Heberlein, *Physician Acceptance of New Medicaid Patients*, Medicaid and CHIP Payment and Access Commission, 2019.

5. Physicians Foundation, "2014 Survey of America's Physicians: Practice Patterns and Perspectives," http://www.physiciansfoundation.org/uploads/default/2014_Physicians_Foundation_Biennial_Physician_Survey_Report.pdf.

6. Commonwealth Fund, "Kaiser Family Foundation/Commonwealth Fund 2015 National Survey of Primary Care Providers," June 2015, https://www.commonwealthfund.org/publications/surveys/2015/jun/kaiser-family-foundationcommonwealth-fund-2015-national-survey.

7. "Opt-Out Affidavits," Centers for Medicare and Medicaid Services, updated November 19, 2019, https://www.cms.gov/Medicare/Provider-Enrollment-and-Certification/MedicareProviderSupEnroll/OptOutAffidavits.

8. J. D. Shatto and M. K. Clemens, "Projected Medicare Expenditures under an Illustrative Scenario with Alternative Payment Updates to Medicare Providers," CMS Office of the Actuary, April 22, 2019.

9. See, for example, M A. Gaglia, "Effect of Insurance Type on Adverse Cardiac Events after Percutaneous Coronary Intervention," *American Journal of*

Cardiology 107 (2011): 675–80; D. J. LaPar et al., "Primary Payer Status Affects Mortality for Major Surgical Operations," *Annals of Surgery* 252 (2010): 544–51; J. Kwok et al., "The Impact of Health Insurance Status on the Survival of Patients with Head and Neck Cancer," *Cancer* 116 (2010): 476–85; R. R. Kelz et al., "Morbidity and Mortality of Colorectal Carcinoma Differs by Insurance Status," *Cancer* 101 (2004): 2187–94; J. G. Allen et al., "Insurance Status Is an Independent Predictor of Long-Term Survival after Lung Transplantation in the United States," *Journal of Heart and Lung Transplantation* 30 (2011): 45–53.

10. Congressional Budget Office, "Insurance Coverage Provisions of the Affordable Care Act—CBO's January 2015 Baseline," https://www.cbo.gov/sites/default/files/cbofiles/attachments/43900-2015-01-ACAtables.pdf.

11. Press release, eHealth, January 3, 2017, https://news.ehealthinsurance.com/news/average-individual-health-insurance-premiums-increased-99-since-2013-the-year-before-obamacare-family-premiums-increased-140-according-to-ehealth-com-shopping-data.

12. "County by County Analysis of Plan Year 2018 Insurer Participation in Health Insurance Exchanges," Centers for Medicare and Medicaid Services, https://www.cms.gov/CCIIO/Programs-and-Initiatives/Health-Insurance-Marketplaces/Downloads/2017-10-20-Issuer-County-Map.pdf.

13. A. Semanskee, G. Claxton, and L. Levitt, "How Premiums Are Changing in 2018," Kaiser Family Foundation, November 29, 2017, https://www.kff.org/health-reform/issue-brief/how-premiums-are-changing-in-2018.

14. Fox and Pickering, "Cost Shift."

15. American Hospital Association and Avalere Health, *Trendwatch Chartbook 2014: Trends Affecting Hospitals and Health Systems* (Washington, DC: American Hospital Association, 2014), http://www.aha.org/research/reports/tw/chartbook/2014/14chartbook.pdf.

16. A. Senger, "Measuring Choice and Competition in the Exchanges: Still Worse Than before the ACA," Heritage Foundation Issue Brief 4324 on Health Care, December 22, 2014, http://www.heritage.org/research/reports/2014/12/measuring-choice-and-competition-in-the-exchanges-still-worse-than-before-the-aca.

17. Congressional Budget Office, *Private Health Insurance and Federal Policy*, February 2016, https://www.cbo.gov/publication/51130.

18. E. Coe et al., "Hospital Networks: Configurations on the Exchanges and Their Impact on Premiums," McKinsey Center for US Health System Reform, December 2013, http://healthcare.mckinsey.com/hospital-networks-configurations-exchanges-and-their-impact-premiums.

19. Avalere Health, "Access to Comprehensive Stroke Centers and Specialty Physicians in Exchange Plans," September 2014, http://www.heart.org/idc/groups/public/@wcm/@adv/documents/downloadable/ucm_468318.pdf.

20. C. F. Pearson , E. Carpenter, and C. Sloan, "Plans with More Restrictive Networks Comprise 73% of Exchange Market," Avalere Health, November 30,

2017, http://avalere.com/expertise/managed-care/insights/plans-with-more
-restrictive-networks-comprise-73-of-exchange-market; "Exchange Plans Include
34 Percent Fewer Providers than the Average for Commercial Plans," Avalere
press release, July 15, 2015, http://avalere.com/expertise/managed-care/insights
/exchange-plans-include-34-percent-fewer-providers-than-the-average-for
-comm.

21. Employer Health Benefits Annual Surveys, 2007–14, Kaiser Family
Foundation, http://kff.org/health-costs/report/employer-health-benefits-annual
-survey-archives.

22. A. Haviland et al., "Do 'Consumer-Directed' Health Plans Bend the Cost
Curve over Time?," NBER Working Paper 21031, National Bureau of Economic
Research, March 2015, http://www.nber.org/papers/w21031.

23. A. Haviland et al., "How Do Consumer-Directed Health Plans Affect
Vulnerable Populations?" *Forum for Health Economics and Policy* 14(2) (2011):
1–12, doi: 10.2202/1558-9544.1248.

24. A. M. Haviland et al., "The Effects of Consumer-Directed Health Plans on
Episodes of Health Care," *Forum for Health Economics and Policy* 14(2) (2011):
1–27, http://www.rand.org/pubs/external_publications/EP201100208.html.

25. S. Wu et al., "Price Transparency for MRIs Increased Use of Less Costly
Providers and Triggered Provider Competition," *Health Affairs* 33 (August 2014):
1391–98, https://doi.org/10.1377/hlthaff.2014.0168; J. C. Robinson, T. Brown, and
C. Whaley, "Reference-Based Benefit Design Changes Consumers' Choices and
Employers' Payments for Ambulatory Surgery," *Health Affairs* 34 (March 2015):
415–22, http://content.healthaffairs.org/content/34/3/415.abstract.

26. Based on my analysis of the Kaiser Family Foundation's employer health
benefits annual survey data, 2006–14; see Kaiser Family Foundation, "Employer
Health Benefits Annual Survey Archives," http://kff.org/health-costs/report
/employer-health-benefits-annual-survey-archives.

27. Edmund F. Haislmaier and Drew Gonshorowski, "Responding to *King v.
Burwell*: Congress's First Step Should Be to Remove Costly Mandates Driving
Up Premiums," Heritage Foundation Issue Brief 4400, May 2015, http://www
.heritage.org/research/reports/2015/05/responding-to-king-v-burwell-congresss
-first-step-should-be-to-remove-costly-mandates-driving-up-premiums; Council for Affordable Health Insurance, *Health Insurance Mandates in the States
2012* (2013), http://www.cahi.org/cahi_contents/resources/pdf/Mandatesin
thestates2012Execsumm.pdf.

28. J. T. O'Connor, "Comprehensive Assessment of ACA Factors That Will
Affect Individual Market Premiums in 2014," *Milliman Reports*, April 25, 2013,
http://ahip.org/MillimanReportACA2013.

29. American Academy of Actuaries, "Drivers of 2016 Health Insurance Premium Changes," Issue Brief, August 2015, http://actuary.org/files/Drivers_2016
_Premiums_080515.pdf.

30. C. Carlson, "Annual Tax on Insurers Allocated by State," *Oliver Wyman Report*, November 2012, http://www.ahip.org/WymanReportNov2012.

31. F. Islami et al., "Proportion and Number of Cancer Cases and Deaths Attributable to Potentially Modifiable Risk Factors in the United States," *CA: A Journal for Clinicians* 68(1) (January 2018): 31–54, doi: 10.3322/caac.21440.

32. B. E. Garrett et al., "Cigarette Smoking: United States, 1965–2008," *Morbidity and Mortality Weekly Report*, January 14, 2011, 109–13.

33. D. Withrow and D. A. Alter, "The Economic Burden of Obesity Worldwide: A Systematic Review of the Direct Costs of Obesity," *Obesity Reviews* 12 (2011): 131–41.

34. R. A. Hammond and R. Levine, "The Economic Impact of Obesity in the United States," *Diabetes, Metabolic Syndrome and Obesity: Targets and Therapy* 3 (2010): 285–95.

35. E. A. Finkelstein et al., "Obesity and Severe Obesity Forecasts through 2030," *American Journal of Preventive Medicine* 42, no. 6 (2012): 563–70, emphasis added.

36. See, for example, J. Wellington, press release, Doermer School of Business and Management Sciences, Indiana University—Purdue University Fort Wayne, 2007; M. Endres et al., "Primary Prevention of Stroke: Blood Pressure, Lipids, and Heart Failure," *European Heart Journal* 32 (2011): 545–55.

37. W. N. Burton et al., "The Economic Costs Associated with Body Mass Index in a Workplace," *Journal of Occupational and Environmental Medicine* 40 (1998): 786–92.

38. Finkelstein et al., "Obesity Forecasts."

39. "Smoking Status and Body Mass Index Relative to Average Individual Health Insurance Premiums," *eHealth* (2011), http://news.ehealthinsurance.com/_ir/68/20125/Smoking_Status_BMI_and_Individual_Health_Insurance_Premiums.pdf.

Chapter 3

1. M. H. Lee, J. D. Schuur, and B. J. Zink, "Owning the Cost of Emergency Medicine: Beyond 2%," *Annals of Emergency Medicine* 62(5) (November 2013): 498–505.

2. D. Pritchard et al., "What Contributes Most to High Health Care Costs? Health Care Spending in High Resource Patients," *Journal of Managed Care and Specialty Pharmacy* 22(2) (February 2016): 102–9; Pharma Evidence, *IMS LifeLink Health Plan Claims Database*, December 2010; Agency for Healthcare Research and Quality, *Medical Expenditure Panel Survey*, 2009.

3. R. A. Cohen and E. P. Zammitti, "High-Deductible Health Plan Enrollment among Adults Aged 18–64 with Employment-Based Insurance Coverage," National Center for Health Statistics Data Brief No. 317, August 2018.

4. Devenir Research, *2018 Year-End HSA Market Statistics and Trends*, February 27, 2019.

5. Testimony Before the Subcommittee on Health of the Ways and Means Committee of the House of Representatives Hearing on Lowering Costs and Expanding Access to Health Care Consumer-Directed Health Plans Submitted by J. L. Dietel, ACFCI, CAS Chief Compliance Officer for WageWorks, Inc., June 6, 2018.

6. A. M. Haviland et al., "The Effects of Consumer-Directed Health Plans.

7. A. M. Haviland et al., "Growth of Consumer-Directed Health Plans to One-Half of All Employer-Sponsored Insurance Could Save $57 Billion Annually," *Health Affairs* 31(5) (2012): 1009–15, http://content.healthaffairs.org/content/31/5/1009.full.

8. National Business Group on Health, *Taking Action to Improve Employee Health: Results from the Sixth Annual Employer-Sponsored Health and Well-Being Survey*, March 25, 2015, https://www.businessgrouphealth.org/pub/29d50202-782b-cb6e-2763-a29a9426f589.

9. Kaiser Family Foundation, *2019 Employer Health Benefits Survey*, September 25, 2019, https://www.kff.org/health-costs/report/2019-employer-health-benefits-survey.

10. Fidelity Investments and the National Business Group on Health, *The Employer Investment in Employee Well-Being: Tenth Annual Employer-Sponsored Health and Well-Being Survey*, 2019.

11. L. L. Berry et al., "What's the Hard Return on Employee Wellness Programs?" *Harvard Business Review*, December 2010, https://hbr.org/2010/12/whats-the-hard-return-on-employee-wellness-programs.

12. K. Baicker et al., "Workplace Wellness Programs Can Generate Savings," *Health Affairs* 29 (2010): 304–11.

Chapter 4

1. B. Stevens, "Blurring the Boundaries: How the Federal Government Has Influenced Welfare Benefits in the Private Sector," in *The Politics of Social Policy in the United States*, eds. M. Weir, A. S. Orloff, and T. Skocpol (Princeton, NJ: Princeton University Press, 1988).

2. P. Starr, *The Social Transformation of American Medicine* (New York: Basic Books, 1982).

3. R. B. Helms, "Tax Policy and the History of the Health Insurance Industry," paper presented at the Taxes and Health Insurance: Analysis and Policy Conference, Brookings Institution, February 29, 2008, http://www.taxpolicycenter.org/tpccontent/healthconference_helms.pdf.

4. S. Lowry, "Itemized Tax Deductions for Individuals: Data Analysis," Congressional Research Service, February 2014, http://www.fas.org/sgp/crs/misc/R43012.pdf.

5. Congressional Budget Office, "Options for Reducing the Deficit: 2014 to 2023," November 2013, http://www.cbo.gov/sites/default/files/cbofiles/attachments /44715-OptionsForReducingDeficit-3.pdf.

6. J. Gruber, "The Tax Exclusion for Employer-Sponsored Health Insurance," *National Tax Journal* 64(2; pt. 2) (June 2011): 511–30.

7. J. Gruber and B. Madrian, "Health Insurance, Labor Supply, and Job Mobility: A Critical Review of the Literature," in *Health Policy and the Uninsured*, ed. C. McLaughlin, 97–108 (Washington, DC: Urban Institute Press, 2004).

8. M. Feldstein and B. Friedman, "Tax Subsidies, the Rational Demand for Insurance and the Health Care Crisis," *Journal of Public Economics* (1977): 155–78.

9. See, for example, A. Finkelstein, "The Aggregate Effects of Health Insurance: Evidence from the Introduction of Medicare," *Quarterly Journal of Economics* 122 (2007): 1–37.

10. I make the assumption that comprehensive tax reform into a broad-based, low-tax-rate system will not likely occur unless compensated in significantly lower overall tax rates and higher after-tax income.

11. Congressional Budget Office, "Options for Reducing the Deficit: 2014 to 2023."

12. Gruber, "Tax Exclusion."

13. L. Clemans-Cope et al., "Limiting the Tax Exclusion of Employer-Sponsored Health Insurance Premiums: Revenue Potential and Distributional Consequences," Robert Wood Johnson Foundation and the Urban Institute, May 2013, http://www.urban.org/sites/default/files/alfresco/publication-pdfs/412816 -Limiting-the-Tax-Exclusion-of-Employer-Sponsored-Health-Insurance -Premiums-Revenue-Potential-and-Distributional-Consequences.PDF.

14. R. Herzlinger and B. D. Richman, *Box 12, IRS W-2, to the Rescue: The Effect of Transferring Pre-Tax Employer-Sponsored Health Insurance Funds to Employees on After-Tax Income, Federal Income and Payroll Taxes, Health Insurance Premiums, and Health Care Costs*, Duke Law School Public Law & Legal Theory Series No. 2019-43, June 18, 2019.

15. Kaiser Family Foundation, *Employer Health Benefit Survey*, 2019.

16. Herzlinger and Richman, *Box 12, IRS W-2, to the Rescue*.

Chapter 5

1. C. Twight, "Medicare's Origin: The Economics and Politics of Dependency," *Cato Journal* 16(3) (1997): 309–38.

2. US Government Accountability Office, "High-Risk Series: An Update," February 2015, 359, http://www.gao.gov/assets/670/668415.pdf.

3. Actuarial data from HealthView using historical claim data and projections, June 2011.

4. J. M. Ortman et al., "An Aging Nation: The Older Population in the United States: Population Estimates and Projection," US Census Bureau Current Population Reports, no. P25-1140, May 2014, https://www.census.gov/prod/2014pubs/p25-1140.pdf.

5. G. Jacobson et al., "Medigap Reform: Setting the Context for Understanding Recent Proposals," Medicare, January 13, 2014, http://kff.org/medicare/issue-brief/medigap-reform-setting-the-context.

6. G. Jacobson et al., *Medicare Advantage 2020 Spotlight: First Look*, Kaiser Family Foundation, October 2019.

7. Author's analysis of Kaiser Family Foundation of *CMS Medicare Advantage Landscape and Enrollment* files, 2010 to 2019.

8. See W. Francis, *Putting Medicare Consumers in Charge: Lessons from the FEHBP* (Washington, DC: AEI Press, 2009).

9. Congressional Budget Office, "Options for Reducing the Deficit: 2014 to 2023."

10. Rebecca Riffkin, "Average U.S. Retirement Age Rises to 62," Gallup, April 2014, http://www.gallup.com/poll/168707/average-retirement-age-rises.aspx.

11. Congressional Budget Office, "Options for Reducing the Deficit: 2014 to 2023"; see especially "Health Revenues—Option 15," 243.

Chapter 6

1. Department of Health and Human Services, "Access to Care: Provider Availability in Medicaid Managed Care," Report OEI-02-13-00670, December 2014, http://oig.hhs.gov/oei/reports/oei-02-13-00670.pdf.

2. See ch. 2 n. 9.

3. A. M. Sisko et al., "National Health Expenditure Projections, 2018–27: Economic and Demographic Trends Drive Spending and Enrollment Growth," *Health Affairs* 38(3) (2019): 491.

4. Congressional Research Service, "Questions about the ACA Medicaid Expansion," memorandum, January 30, 2015, https://www.heartland.org/sites/default/files/crs_memo_-_questions_about_the_aca_medicaid_expansion_-_jan_2015.pdf.

5. Pritchard et al., "High Health Care Costs."

Chapter 7

1. L. Dafny, "Hospital Industry Consolidation—Still More to Come?" *New England Journal of Medicine* 370 (2014): 198–99, doi: 10.1056/NEJMp1313948.

2. M. Gaynor, F. Mostashari, and P. B. Ginsburg, "Making Health Care Markets Work: Competition Policy for Health Care," *JAMA* 317(13) (2017): 1313–14.

3. M. Gaynor and R. Town, *The Impact of Hospital Consolidation*, Robert Wood Johnson Foundation, June 1, 2012, https://www.rwjf.org/en/library /research/2012/06/the-impact-of-hospital-consolidation.html.

4. J. C. Robinson and K. Miller, "Total Expenditures per Patient in Hospital-Owned and Physician-Owned Physician Organizations in California," *JAMA* 312(16) (2014): 1663–69, doi: 10.1001/jama.2014.14072.

5. C. Capps, D. Dranove, and C. Ody, *The Effect of Hospital Acquisitions of Physician Practices on Prices and Spending*, Working Paper Series WP-15-02, Institute for Policy Research, Northwestern University, February 2015.

6. J. S. Ashwood et al., "Trends in Retail Clinic Use among the Commercially Insured," *American Journal of Managed Care* 17(11) (2011): e443–48.

7. A. Mehrotra et al., "The Costs and Quality of Care for Three Common Illnesses at Retail Clinics as Compared to Other Medical Settings," *Annals of Internal Medicine* 151(5) (2009): 321–28.

8. R. M. Weinick et al., "Policy Implications of the Use of Retail Clinics," Rand Health Technical Report, 2010, http://www.rand.org/content/dam/rand /pubs/technical_reports/2010/RAND_TR810.pdf.

9. Accenture, "Retail Medical Clinics Will Double between 2012 and 2015 and Save $800 Million per Year," June 2013, https://www.accenture.com/_acnme dia/Accenture/Conversion-Assets/DotCom/Documents/Global/PDF/Dual pub_21/Accenture-Retail-Medical-Clinics-From-Foe-to-Friend.pdf.

10. Blue Cross Blue Shield, *Retail Clinic Visits Increase Despite Use Lagging among Individually Insured Americans*, Health of America report, 2016.

11. R. Rudavsky et al., "The Geographic Distribution, Ownership, Prices, and Scope of Practice at Retail Clinics," *Annals of Internal Medicine* 151 (2009): 315–20.

12. T. Yee, E. Boukus, D. Cross, and D. Samuel, *Primary Care Workforce Shortages: Nurse Practitioner Scope-of-Practice Laws and Payment Policies*, National Institute for Health Care Reform Research Brief no. 13, February 2013.

13. Committee on the Robert Wood Foundation Initiative on the Future of Nursing, *The Future of Nursing: Leading Change, Advancing Health* (Washington, DC: National Academies Press, 2011), http://www.nap.edu/catalog/12956 /the-future-of-nursing-leading-change-advancing-health.

14. Association of American Medical Colleges, "The Complexities of Physician Supply and Demand: Projections through 2025," Report of the Center for Workforce Studies, 2008, https://members.aamc.org/eweb/upload/The%20Complexities %20of%20Physician%20Supply.pdf.

15. Centers for Disease Control and Prevention/National Center for Health Statistics, *Population Aging and the Use of Office-Based Physician Services*, NCHS Data Brief no. 41, August 2010, http://www.cdc.gov/nchs/data/databriefs /db41.PDF; Centers for Disease Control, *National Ambulatory Medical Care Survey*, 1978 and 2008.

16. "CON—Certificate of Need State Laws, " National Conference of State Legislatures, August 25, 2016, http://www.ncsl.org/research/health/con-certi ficate-of-need-state-laws.aspx.

17. J. A. DiMasi, H. G. Grabowski, and R. W. Hansen, "Innovation in the Pharmaceutical Industry: New Estimates of R&D Costs," Tufts Center for the Study of Drug Development, R&D Cost Study Briefing, Boston, November 18, 2014; F. Pammolli et al., "The Productivity Crisis in Pharmaceutical R&D," *Nature Reviews Drug Discovery* 10 (2011): 428–38.

18. J. Makower et al., "FDA Impact on US Medical Technology Innovation," November 2010, http://eucomed.org/uploads/Press%20Releases/FDA%20impact% 20on%20U.S.%20Medical%20Technology%20Innovation.pdf.

19. National Community Pharmacists Association News Release, "Pharmacists Survey: Prescription Drug Costs Skewed by Fees on Pharmacies, Patients," June 28, 2016; K. Van Nuys et al., "Frequency and Magnitude of Co-payments Exceeding Prescription Drug Costs," *JAMA* 319(10) (2018): 1045–47, doi: 10.1001/jama.2018.0102.

20. Credit Suisse, *Global Pharmaceuticals and Biotechnology*, April 18, 2017.

21. F. de Brantes and S. Delbanco, *Report Card on State Price Transparency Laws*, Health Care Incentives Improvement Institute, July 2016.

22. A. Higgins, N. Brainard, and G. Veselovskiy, "Characterizing Health Plan Price Estimator Tools: Findings from a National Survey," *American Journal of Managed Care* 22(2) (2016): 126–31.

23. Y.-C. Shih, S. Fuld Nasso, and S. Yousuf Zafa, "Price Transparency for Whom? In Search of Out-of-Pocket Cost Estimates to Facilitate Cost Communication in Cancer Care," *PharmacoEconomics* 36 (2018): 259–61.

24. I. Cockburn, J. O. Lanjouw, and M. Schankerman, "Patents and the Global Diffusion of New Drugs," *American Economic Review* 106(1) (2016): 136–64.

25. "Shop Around for Lower Drug Prices," *Consumer Reports*, April 5, 2018, https://www.consumerreports.org/drug-prices/shop-around-for-better-drug -prices.

26. Cornell University, INSEAD, and WIPO, *The Global Innovation Index 2019: Creating Healthy Lives—the Future of Medical Innovation, Ithaca, Fontainebleau, and Geneva*, 2019.

27. "2014 Global R&D Funding Forecast," Battelle and *R&D Magazine*, https://www.battelle.org/docs/tpp/2014_global_rd_funding_forecast.pdf.

28. C. J. Charkesworth, E. Smit, D. S. Lee, F. Alramadhan, and M. C. Odden, "Polypharmacy Among Adults Aged 65 Years and Older in the United States: 1988–2010," *The Journals of Gerontology. Series A, Biological Sciences and Medical Sciences* 70, no. 8 (August 2015): 989–95, https://academic.oup.com/bio medgerontology/article/70/8/989/2947682.

29. IQVIA Institute for Human Data Science, "Medicine Use and Spending in the US: A Review of 2018 and Outlook to 2023," Institute Report, May 9,

2019, https://www.iqvia.com/insights/the-iqvia-institute/reports/medicine-use
-and-spending-in-the-us-a-review-of-2018-and-outlook-to-2023.

30. John Elflein, "Percentage of Older People Who Received an Influenza
Vaccination during the Past 12 Months in the U.S. from 1997 to 2018," Statista,
https://www.statista.com/statistics/244615/share-of-us-persons-who-received
-an-influenza-vaccination.

31. John Elflein, "Percentage of U.S. College Students That Had Received
Select Vaccinations as of fall 2018," Statista; https://www.statista.com/statistics
/826994/vaccination-coverage-among-us-college-students.

32. John Elflein, "Percentage of Children Aged 19-35 Months Who Are Vac-
cinated against Measles, Mumps And Rubella (MMR) in the U.S. from 1994 to
2017," Statista, https://www.statista.com/statistics/385577/mmr-vaccination-rate
-among-us-children-aged-19-35-months.

33. "Are Generic Drugs Like Apotex Medication Made in India Safe?," Consumer Reports, April 25, 2014, https://www.consumerreports.org/cro/news/2014
/04/are-generic-drugs-made-in-india-safe/index.htm.

34. US Government Accountability Office, "Drug Safety: Preliminary Findings Indicate Persistent Challenges with FDA Foreign Inspections," Statement
of Mary Denigan-Macauley, Director, Health Care, GAO-20-262T, December 10, 2019, https://www.gao.gov/assets/710/703078.pdf.

35. Curtis Dombeck, "Federal Circuit Revolutionizes Country of Origin
Analysis for Pharmaceuticals," FDA Law Update, Sheppard Mullin, February 11, 2020, https://www.fdalawblog.com/2020/02/articles/enforcement
-actions/country-of-origin-analysis-pharmaceuticals.

36. William L. Hamilton, Cormac Doyle, Mycroft Halliwell-Ewen, and
Gabriel Lambert, "Public Health Interventions to Protect against Falsified
Medicines: A Systematic Review of International, National and Local Policies,"
Health Policy and Planning, 31, no. 10 (December 2016):, 1448–66; https://doi.org
/10.1093/heapol/czw062.

37. US Food and Drug Administration, "FDA Announces Voluntary Recall
of Several Medicines Containing Valsartan Following Detection of an Impurity," FDA News Release, July 13, 2018, https://www.fda.gov/news-events/press
-announcements/fda-announces-voluntary-recall-several-medicines-containing
-valsartan-following-detection-impurity.

38. US Food and Drug Administration, "Information on Heparin," February 5,
2018, https://www.fda.gov/drugs/postmarket-drug-safety-information-patients
-and-providers/information-heparin.

39. Javier C. Hernández, "In China, Vaccine Scandal Infuriates Parents and
Tests Government," New York Times, July 23, 2018.

40. Paul N Newton, Patricia Tabernero, Prabha Dwivedi, María J Culzoni,
María Eugenia Monge, Isabel Swamidoss, Dallas Mildenhall, et al., "Falsified
Medicines in Africa: All Talk, No Action," *Lancet Global Health* 2, no. 9
(September 2014): e509–10, https://core.ac.uk/download/pdf/29050217.pdf.

41. US Food and Drug Administration, "Generic Drug Facts," June 1, 2018, https://www.fda.gov/drugs/generic-drugs /generic-drug-facts.

42. US Government Accountability Office, "Drug Safety."

43. US Food and Drug Administration, "Imported Drugs Raise Safety Concerns," March 1, 2018, https://www.fda.gov/drugs/drug-information-consumers /imported-drugs-raise-safety-concerns.

44. Robert Kneller, "The Importance of New Companies for Drug Discovery: Origins of a Decade of New Drugs," *Nature Reviews Drug Discovery* 9, no. 11 (November 2010): 867–82, https://www.nature.com/articles/nrd3251.pdf.

45. Daniel Workman, "Drugs and Medicine Exports by Country, World's Top Exports, April 25, 2020, http://www.worldstopexports.com/drugs-medicine -exports-country.

46. Matej Mikulic, "Availability of New Cancer Drugs Launched in 2013–2017 in Selected Countries as of 2018," Statista, https://www.statista.com/statistics /696020/availability-of-new-oncology-drugs-by-country.

47. Wanqing Chen, Rongshou Zheng, Peter D. Baade, Siwei Zhang, Hongmei Zeng, Freddie Bray, Ahmedin Jemal, Xue Qin Yu, and Jie He, "Cancer Statistics in China, 2015," *CA: A Cancer Journal for Clinicians*, 66, no. 2 (March/April 2016): 115–32, https://acsjournals.onlinelibrary.wiley.com/doi/full/10.3322/caac .21338.

48. Hongmei Zeng, Rongshou Zheng, Yuming Guo, Siwei Zhang, Xiaonong Zou, Ning Wang, Limei Zhang, et al., "Cancer Survival in China, 2003–2005: A Population-Based Study," *International Journal of Cancer* 136, no. 8 (April 15, 2015): 1921–30, https://onlinelibrary.wiley.com/doi/full/10.1002/ijc.29227.

49. "Zero Percent Import Tariffs on Common and Cancer Drugs in China," Official announcement by the State Council of the People's Republic of China, https://acolink.com/news/2018/import-tarrif-reduced-to-zero-on-common -drugs.

50. World Intellectual Property Organization, "Statistical Country Profiles," accessed April 2020, https://www.wipo.int/ipstats/en/statistics/country_profile.

51. Mary Jo Lamberti and Kenneth Getz, "Profiles of New Approaches to Improving the Efficiency and Performance of Pharmaceutical Drug Development," Tufts Center for the Study of Drug Development White Paper, May 2015, https://csdd.tufts.edu/s/CSSD_PhRMAWhitePaperNEWEST2.pdf.

52. Kenneth Getz, "Trends Driving Clinical Trials into Large Clinical Care Settings," *Nature Reviews Drug Discovery* 17, no. 10 (October 2018): 703–4, https://doi.org/10.1038/nrd.2018.111.

53. US Executive Office of the President, Council of Economic Advisers, *Measuring Prescription Drug Prices: A Primer on the CPI Prescription Drug Index*, October 2019, https://www.whitehouse.gov/wp-content/uploads/2019/10 /Measuring-Prescription-Drug-Prices-A-Primer-on-the-CPI-Prescription-Drug -Index.pdf.

54. Rexford E. Santerre and John A. Vernon, "Assessing Consumer Gains from a Drug Price Control Policy in the United States," *Southern Economic Journal* 73, no. 1 (July 2006) 233–45, http://www.nber.org/papers/w11139.

55. Iain M. Cockburn, Jean O. Lanjouw, and Mark Schankerman, "Patents and the Global Diffusion of New Drugs," *American Economic Review* 106, no. 1 (January 2016): 136–64, http://www.nber.org/papers/w20492.

56. Thomas A. Abbott and John A. Vernon, "The Cost of US Pharmaceutical Price Regulation: A Financial Simulation Model of R&D Decisions," *Managerial and Decision Economics* 28, no. 4–5 (June–August 2007): 293–306, https://www.nber.org/papers/w11114.

57. Council of Economic Advisers, *Reforming Biopharmaceutical Pricing at Home and Abroad*, February 2018.

58. Cockburn, Lanjouw, and Schankerman, "Patents and the Global Diffusion."

59. R. E. Santerre and J. A. Vernon, "Assessing Consumer Gains from a Drug Price Control Policy in the United States," *Southern Economic Journal* 73 (2006): 233–45.

60. US Senator Bernie Sanders, The Prescription Drug Price Relief Act of 2019, https://www.sanders.senate.gov/download/final_-prescription-drug-price-relief-act-of-2019---summary?id=D3922119-B92C-41F0-997D-2B931E34B2FE&download=1&inline=file.

61. National Institute for Health and Care Excellence, *Changes to NICE Drug Appraisals: What You Need to Know*, NHS England, April 4, 2017, https://www.nice.org.uk/news/feature/changes-to-nice-drug-appraisals-what-you-need-to-know.

62. M. M. Mello et al., "National Costs of the Medical Liability System," *Health Affairs* 29 (2010): 1569–77.

63. V. Wadhwa, *The Immigrant Exodus: Why America Is Losing the Global Race to Capture Entrepreneurial Talent* (Philadelphia: Wharton Digital Press, 2012).

Q&A

1. M. Frean, J. Gruber, and B. D. Sommers, "Disentangling the ACA's Coverage Effects—Lessons for Policymakers," *New England Journal of Medicine* 375(17) (2016): 1605–08.

2. J. Hadley et al., "Covering the Uninsured in 2008: Current Costs, Sources of Payment, and Incremental Costs," *Health Affairs* 27(suppl. 1) (2008): w399–w415, https://doi.org/10.1377/hlthaff.27.5.w399.

3. T. A. Coughlin et al., "Uncompensated Care for Uninsured in 2013," Kaiser Family Foundation, May 2014.

4. K. Baicker et al., "The Oregon Experiment—Effects of Medicaid on Clinical Outcomes," *New England Journal of Medicine* 368(18) (2013): 1713–22.

5. J. T. O'Connor, "ACA Factors."

6. See White House, *Analytical Perspectives: Budget of the US Government, Fiscal Year 2016*, Office of Management and Budget, 255.

7. See N. Brennan and M. Shepard, "Comparing Quality of Care in the Medicare Program," *American Journal of Managed Care* 16(11) (2010): 841–48.

8. J. S. Guram and R. E. Moffit, "The Medicare Advantage Success Story—Looking beyond the Cost Difference," *New England Journal of Medicine* 366(13) (2012): 1177–79.

9. R. W. Fairlie, "Immigrant Entrepreneurs and Small Business Owners, and their Access to Financial Capital," Small Business Administration, Office of Advocacy, 2012

10. "The Economic Case for Welcoming Immigrant Entrepreneurs," *Entrepreneurship Policy Digest*, Kauffman Foundation, March 27, 2014; updated September 8, 2015.

About the Author

Scott W. Atlas, MD, is the Robert Wesson Senior Fellow in Scientific Philosophy and Public Policy at Stanford University's Hoover Institution and a member of Hoover's Working Group on Health Care Policy. He investigates the impact of government and the private sector on access, quality, and pricing; global trends in health care innovation; and key economic issues related to the future of technology-based medical advances. Dr. Atlas is a frequent policy adviser to policy makers and government officials. He has served as senior adviser for health care to a number of candidates for president of the United States. He often travels to Washington, DC, to testify before Congressional committees and conduct policy briefings on Capitol Hill and for the directors of key agencies in the federal government. Dr. Atlas's most recent books, in addition to the first edition of *Restoring Quality Health Care* (Hoover Institution Press, 2016), include *In Excellent Health: Setting the Record Straight on America's Health Care System* (Hoover Institution Press, 2011), and *Reforming America's Health Care System* (Hoover Institution Press, 2010). His work and interviews have appeared worldwide, in media including BBC Radio, *PBS NewsHour*, the *Wall Street Journal*, the *New York Times*, *The Hill*, *Forbes*, CNN, *USA Today*, Fox News, London's *Financial Times*, Brazil's *Isto E*, Italy's *Corriere della Sera*, Argentina's *Diario La Nación*, and India's *The Hindu*. Dr. Atlas also advises entrepreneurs and companies in the life sciences, medical technology, and health information technology sectors.

Dr. Atlas is also the editor of *Magnetic Resonance Imaging of the Brain and Spine*, the leading textbook in the field, which has been translated from English into Mandarin, Spanish, and Portuguese and is in its fifth edition. He has been an editor, an associate editor, and a member of the editorial and scientific boards of several journals as well as national and international scientific societies during the past three decades. As professor and chief of neuroradiology at Stanford University Medical Center from 1998 until 2012 and during his prior academic positions, Dr. Atlas trained more than one hundred neuroradiology fellows, many of whom are now leaders in the field throughout the world. Dr. Atlas is recognized internationally as a leader in both education and clinical research and has received numerous awards and honors in recognition of his leadership in these fields.

Dr. Atlas received a BS degree in biology from the University of Illinois in Urbana-Champaign and an MD degree from the University of Chicago School of Medicine.

Index